From Calcedonies to Orchids:

Plays Promoting Humanity in Health Policy

From Calcedonies to Orchids:

Plays Promoting Humanity in Health Policy

Jeff Nisker

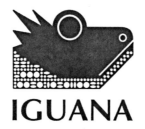

IGUANA

Published by Iguana Books
460 Richmond St. West, Suite 401
Toronto, Ontario, Canada
M5V 1Y1

Publisher: Greg Ioannou
Front cover image: Jeff Nisker
Front cover design: Jane Awde Goodwin
Book layout and design: Stephanie Martin

Library and Archives Canada Cataloguing in Publication

Nisker, Jeffrey A.
     From Calcedonies to Orchids : plays promoting humanity in health policy / Jeff Nisker.

Contents: Calcedonies -- Sarah's daughters -- A child on her mind -- Camouflage -- Philip -- Orchids.
Issued also in electronic formats.
ISBN 978-1-927403-36-5

     I. Title.

PS8627.I85F76 2013   C812'.6   C2012-908569-3

This is the original print edition of *From Calcedonies to Orchids: Plays Promoting Humanity in Health Policy.*

To the women who made this book possible.

Table of Contents

Introduction

Humanity, it seems, is being systematically supplanted in ethics deliberations to create health policies. Accountability to the humanity of the persons immersed in health policy issues is being dissolved in the red ink of accountability to supposedly "fixed" health funding, too often fixated on the black ink of quantifiable "metrics of care," such as patients through the turnstile and the cost-effectiveness of survival strategy. Parameters such as wellness, respect, dignity, and compassion, being more difficult for a computer to calculate, are bottom-line ignored.

Theatre can help humanity re-emerge as the primary imperative of health policy deliberation by encouraging audience members to approximate empathy for persons too often invisible to health policy makers, too often different from ourselves, but not really. The simultaneous exploration of issues of health policy ethics and humanity through theatre encourages us to see the uniqueness and beauty of each person, no matter how rampant or difficult the problems they face.[1] Indeed, though I completed *Orchids* in 1995 and *Calcedonies* in 2011, the plays are presented "*From Calcedonies to Orchids*" because we first need to see the beautiful calcedony that is each person, beneath the medicalized layers of illness and difference, before we can cultivate a culture that will promote the flourishing of those who require care or accommodation, as is required for *Orchids*.

During and resulting from the many interviews I conducted for these plays, I experienced and learned much that I hope to convey to you in these pages. Writing plays is the best way I know to explore ethical issues of health policies and to promote compassionate decisions by health policy makers, for policy makers must be accountable to the public.

So how did a clinician and scientist come to believe that theatre could promote humanity in health policy deliberation and ultimately in health promotion and care? As a teenager, between medical school boot camps, I worked at a summer camp, where, in addition to helping the children swim and canoe, I wrote camp-centred takeoffs of Broadway musicals for the campers and staff to perform. Writing these primitive adaptations saved me from total consumption in the miles of medical

---

[1] J. Nisker, Health-policy research and the possibilities of theatre, in J.G. Knowles and A.L. Cole (eds.), *Handbook of the Arts in Qualitative Research: Perspectives, Methodologies, Examples, and Issues.* Thousand Oaks, CA: Sage Publications, 2008, pp. 613–624.

ink[2] that had rapidly dissolved my addiction to literature. But medical school graduation marked the end of my summers of plays.

During my specialty training,[3] I began researching the relationship of estrogen to cancer.[4] This research resulted in a Medical Research Council of Canada fellowship to work in a laboratory in California, where I spent much of my time zipped into my Canadian winter jacket, as my research required working in a large refrigerator. We found that continuous high levels of biologically free estrogen caused uterine cancer and possibly breast cancer. The more we found, the farther theatre faded.[5]

On my return to Canada,[6] I continued my research in a laboratory adjacent to the hospital where I cared for women with these cancers. We were fortunate to find that rabbits naturally developed the same kind of uterine cancer as women because they also had high continuous biologically free estrogen levels. After five years of a randomized research trial, we found that rabbit uterine cancer could be prevented by anti-estrogens.[7] However, as my clinical practice and my family grew, I had less and less time for research, let alone writing plays. But the convergence of three streams[8] would soon lead me back to theatre, and, melded with my research training, would help me to write *Orchids* and *Sarah's Daughters*; melded with my clinical training, would help me to write *A Child on Her Mind* and *Philip*; and melded with my good fortune of wonderful directors, would help me to dig deeper within myself to write *Calcedonies* and *Camouflage*.

---

[2] J.A. Nisker, The yellow brick road of medical education, *Canadian Medical Association Journal*, 1997, 156, 689–691.
[3] J. Nisker, Theatre and Research in the Reproductive Sciences, *Journal of Medical Humanities*, 2010, 31(1), 81-90.
[4] I. Ramzy and J.A. Nisker, Histologic study of ovaries from young women with endometrial adenocarcinoma, *American Journal of Clinical Pathology*, 1979, 71(3), 253–256; J.A. Nisker, I. Ramzy, and J. A. Collins, Adenocarcinoma of the endometrium and abnormal ovarian function in young women, *American Journal of Obstetrics and Gynecology*, 1978, 130(5), 546–550.
[5] J.A. Nisker, G.L. Hammond, B.J. Davidson, A.M. Frumar, N. K. Takaki, H L. Judd, and P.K. Siiteri, Serum sex hormone-binding globulin capacity and the percentage of free estradiol in postmenopausal women with and without endometrial carcinoma: A new biochemical basis for the association between obesity and endometrial carcinoma, *American Journal of Obstetrics and Gynecology*, 1980, 138(6), 637–642.
[6] J. Nisker, Theatre and Research in the Reproductive Sciences, *Journal of Medical Humanities*, 2010, 31(1), 81-90.
[7] J.A. Nisker, M.E. Kirk, and J.T. Nunez-Troconis, Reduced incidence of rabbit endometrial neoplasia with levonorgestrel implant, *American Journal of Obstetrics and Gynecology*, 1988, 158(2), 300–303.
[8] The three streams are discussed in J. Nisker, Theatre and research in the reproductive sciences, *Journal of Medical Humanities*, 2010, 31, 81–90.

The first stream[9] was genetic science, which became torrential in the 1987 downstream of Kary Mullis's Nobel prize–winning production of the "polymerase chain reaction."[10] This chain reaction allowed the rapid million-fold multiplication of DNA and caused chain reactions throughout science by giving each of us a bright new hammer with which we, of course, sought something that "looks like a nail."[11] The nail I was sent to seek was the possibility of genetic testing of in vitro fertilized embryos, so-called preimplantation genetic diagnosis (PGD). Our aim was to offer to women the obviation of both amniocentesis at sixteen weeks of pregnancy and consideration of termination weeks later when they received the results. After I had been researching PGD on mouse embryos for two years, a woman undergoing in vitro fertilization (IVF) at University Hospital told one of the nurses that if she became pregnant she planned to have amniocentesis because she carried a gene for a serious genetic condition. With our university's research ethics board approval, and with an extensive informed choice process (if, as Susan Sherwin[12] and Françoise Baylis[13] point out, informed choice is ever possible regarding IVF), we offered this woman PGD in a research setting. She decided to pursue this route and we performed Canada's first PGD. The next day, someone leaked this news, and Canada's national media networks descended upon me. My office was deluged with calls from across Canada, from prospective parents requesting PGD. I had been warned by my friends in the feminist movement, most strongly by Abby Lippman of the Council of Responsible Genetics, that PGD was an inappropriate focus of research for a feminist like me. I rebutted that "slippery slopes could be melted by sensitive scientists"; but when more than half of the requests for PGD were to avoid the genetic condition of the XX chromosome (a girl), I stopped my research program, wrote my concerns, which were published in a clinical journal for physicians' consideration,[14] and began writing *Orchids*[15] for public consideration (and as a mea culpa to my feminist friends).

---

[9] J. Nisker, Theatre and Research in the Reproductive Sciences, *Journal of Medical Humanities*, 2010, 31(1), 81-90.

[10] K.B. Mullis and F. Faloona, Specific synthesis of DNA in vitro via a polymerase-catalyzed chain reaction, *Methods in Enzymology*, 1987, 155, 335–350.

[11] Phish, "Bittersweet Motel," M.E. Gordon and P. McConnell (songwriters), in T. Phillips (dir.), *Bittersweet Motel*, DVD, Los Angeles: Image Entertainment, 2001.

[12] S. Sherwin, *No Longer Patient: Feminist Ethics and Health Care*. Philadelphia: Temple University Press, 1992.

[13] F.E. Baylis, The ethics of ex utero research on spare 'non-viable' IVF human embryos, *Bioethics*, 1990, 4(4), 311–329.

[14] J.A. Nisker and R.E. Gore-Langton, Pre-implantation genetic diagnosis: A model of progress and concern, *Journal of Obstetrics and Gynaecology Canada*, 1995, 17(3), 247–262.

[15] J.A. Nisker, Orchids: Not necessarily a gospel, in J. Murray (ed.), *Mappa Mundi: Mapping Culture/Mapping the World*, Windsor, ON: University of Windsor Press, 2001, pp. 61–109.

The sources of the second stream were the funding cutbacks to both higher education and hospitals,[16] resulting from our newly elected government's fulfillment of its promise of personal income tax breaks. Our university's bioethics institute was an early fatality, as it was funded equally by the university and the teaching hospitals, and ethics is frequently the first casualty of cutbacks. After the ethics institute's philosopher-ethicists relocated, my Dean, who must have thought that I could teach bioethics given my worries regarding PGD, asked me to take over bioethics teaching. Fortunately, the third stream,[17] my children's bedtime stories, merged with the other two before I could reply with the unequivocal "yes" one usually replies to one's Dean.

Every night, I would read to my pyjama'd children what one of their sleepover friends termed "The Thought for the Night" (which was really a shameless washing of young minds toward social justice thinking[18]). One night, on the advice of a colleague, I read from a book with which I was unfamiliar, *The Little Prince* by Antoine de St. Exupéry.[19] I came to the line where the fox advises the Little Prince that, "It is only with the heart that one can see rightly for what is essential is invisible to the eye," and I must have read it over and over, as one of my children finally asked, "Are you okay Dad?" I promptly responded, "It's time to go to sleep." I knew I had read something epiphanic and needed time to consider what it meant. Over that night, I came to understand that we needed to explore health ethics with our hearts, rather than just applying principles and theories with the same multiple-choice objectivity we medical types are taught to use when cognating symptoms and signs of disease.[20] So when my Dean asked me to take over the bioethics curriculum, I responded with a "yes-but," only if I could use theatre to engage the students' hearts as well as their minds.

In the health ethics and humanities program we started in 1995, each three-hour exploration begins with a play or a "readers' theatre" of a poem or short story,[21] upon which is based the ensuing discussion of

---

[16] J. Nisker, Theatre and Research in the Reproductive Sciences, *Journal of Medical Humanities*, 2010, 31(1), 81-90.
[17] J. Nisker, Theatre and Research in the Reproductive Sciences, *Journal of Medical Humanities*, 2010, 31(1), 81-90.
[18] J. Nisker, Preface, in J. Nisker (ed.), *From the Other Side of the Fence: Stories from Health Care Professionals*, Halifax: Pottersfield Press, 2008, pp. 11–15.
[19] A. de Saint-Exupéry, *The Little Prince*, San Diego: Harcourt Brace Jovanovich, 1943.
[20] J.A. Nisker, The yellow brick road of medical education, *Canadian Medical Association Journal*, 1997, 156, 689–691; J.A. Nisker, Narrative ethics in health care, in J.P. Storch, P. Rodney and R. Starzomski (eds.), *Toward a Moral Horizon: Nursing Ethics for Leadership and Practice*, Toronto: Pearson Prentice Hall, 2004, pp. 285–310; J. Nisker, Theatre and Research in the Reproductive Sciences, *Journal of Medical Humanities*, 2010, 31(1), 81-90.
[21] "Readers' theatre," Centre of Literature and Medicine, 1996

health policy or professionalism. I found this progression promoted empathy for the persons in the centre of the health ethics issue, rather than objectifying complex issues in multiple-choice, short-answer, or other exam-efficient formats. I saw excitement in medical students' eyes, not the ethics-eyelid reflex of which I had been forewarned. I was convinced that theatre-based programs for medical students (and indeed physicians) would protect their hearts from succumbing to medical education's over-objectivity. I was also convinced that theatre would be useful for the more compassion-considering health professions such as nursing and for the general public, to involve them, through their voices and votes, in compassionate health policy development.[22]

In writing science-based plays for the general public, it is essential that audience members be provided with the necessary scientific and clinical information in an easily digestible manner, while at the same time engaging them in the position of the characters in the vortex of the issue being explored. Both can be accomplished through dialogue between characters, as in *Orchids* and *A Child on Her Mind*; in dialogues between the central characters and the audience as in *Sarah's Daughters*, *Camouflage*, and *Calcedonies*; or even through a mock lecture as was necessary for conveying the complex genetic information in *Sarah's Daughters*. To permit my plays to be seen by more people, of more diverse perspectives, in more geographic regions, I am increasingly drawn to writing plays for one or two actors, with minimal sets, as in *Sarah's Daughters* and as is planned for *Calcedonies* and *Camouflage*, rather than the six actors in *A Child on Her Mind* or the four leads and a chorus in *Orchids*. The more people theatre engages, the more likely compassionate health policy will occur.

Theatre has been used to engage the public in social issues since Ancient Greece, and probably earlier. Shakespeare explored social issues. Schiller's *Wilhelm Tell* promoted democracy in 14th-century Europe,[23] and Boal's plays taught democracy in the Brazil of the 1960s and 1970s. Boal describes his work as "theatre helping to bring about social transformation" and believes that theatre accomplishes such transformation by allowing us to be "simultaneously Protagonist and principal spectator of our actions."[24] Martha Nussbaum writes that the

---

[22] J. Nisker, Preface, in J. Nisker (ed.), *From the Other Side of the Fence: Stories from Health Care Professionals*, Halifax, NS: Pottersfield Press, 2008, pp. 11–15.

[23] E. Batley and D. Bradby, Introduction, in E. Batley and D. Bradby (eds.), *Morality and Justice: The Challenge of European Theatre*, special issue of *European Studies*, 2001, 17, Amsterdam: Rodopi Bv Editions, pp. 11–12.

[24] A. Boal, *Legislative Theatre: Using Performance to Make Politics*, London: Routledge, 1998.

theatre audience member "makes sense of the suffering by recognizing that one might oneself encounter such a reversal."[25]

In the plays included in this book, I have tried to help audience members identify with the central characters, rather than just analyze the health policy issue. This was most difficult and is most important in *Calcedonies*. *Calcedonies* is a work of fiction built on true occurrences in the life of a woman who asked me to write a play about her to expose the injustices inflicted upon disabled persons by Canada's supposedly wonderful health and social support systems.[26] *Calcedonies* is my attempt to engage the public in discussion of these injustices and to change the systems that let this wonderful woman down. Change can happen only when equality rather than cost-effectiveness, fairness rather than finance, once again become prevailing imperatives. *Calcedonies* also includes a true occurrence with my friend Catherine Frazee, a well-known writer and disabilities activist. Catherine's inspiration and kindness is imbued throughout *Calcedonies*.

Sarah's Daughters explores the anguish of a young woman whose mother and grandmother died of hereditary breast cancer in their forties and "who lives with the knowledge it will happen to her."[27] Again based on true stories, and again drawing attention to unjust health policy, *Sarah's Daughters* issues tells the story of woman at very high risk of developing hereditary breast cancer denied access to genetic counselling, cancer genetics testing, and cancer prevention strategies. *Sarah's Daughters* also begins a conversation toward compassionate appreciation of genetic risk and sensitive understanding of its consequences. The play argues that as genetic knowledge infiltrates our lives, it will not be submerged by secrets and lies that cause worry about developing cancer and fear of genetic discrimination. *Sarah's Daughters* offers a way for the love inherent in a multi-generational family to soothe the truth of a terrible disease and promote strategies for its prevention. The play has been performed in five countries.

Through the stories of three women, their labour coaches, and the nurse that helps them through labour, A Child on Her Mind examines the disparate realities of becoming a mother amid societal pressures, socioeconomic and age limitations, and new reproductive technologies.[28]

[25] M.C. Nussbaum, *Upheavals of Thought: The Intelligence of Emotions*, Cambridge, UK: Cambridge University Press, 2001, p. 316.
[26] J. Nisker, Calcedonies: Critical reflections on writing plays to engage citizens in health and social policy development. *Reflective Practice: International and Multidisciplinary Perspectives*, 2010, 11(4), 417–432.
[27] J. Nisker, She lived with the knowledge, *Ars Medica*, 2004, 1(1), 75–80.
[28] J. Nisker, Introduction to A Child on Her Mind, in V. Bergum, J. Van Der Zalm (eds.), *Mother Life: Studies of Mothering Experience*, Edmonton, AB: Pedagon Publishing, 2007, pp. 358–363.

I wrote *A Child on Her Mind* as a result of the media coverage of Orchids. Vangie Bergum, a Professor of Nursing and Health Ethics at the University of Alberta, had heard about Orchids and asked me to write a play based on her book. *A Child on Her Mind: The Experience of Becoming a Mother.*[29] Vangie's writing (from her PhD thesis research) provided the "warp" on which I could weave my research and concerns regarding the exploitation of socioeconomically disadvantaged women in egg "sharing," "bartering," and "donation,"[30] and also regarding acting as surrogate mothers.[31] I wanted to bring to the public the complex concepts emerging in our society, which was increasingly being exposed to both assisted reproduction and social inequality. *A Child on Her Mind* juxtaposes the beauty of becoming a mother with the ugliness spawned by inequality of access to new reproductive technology, societal impellations, socio-economic inequalities, and relationship differentials. *A Child on Her Mind* surfaces the reproductive coercion arising from emerging technology, and the socio-economic prejudices that foster coercion.[32]

Through *Camouflage*, I hope to stimulate public discussion among health professionals and the public regarding the often ignored health promotion issue of intimate partner violence. The harm is particularly ignored when no physical bruises provide clues to the chronic violation. *Camouflage* is based on two personal stories relating how I could have possibly done more to prevent such violence and to provide care for women confined in a house of psychological violence. *Camouflage* also includes parts of a short story by Kathleen Tomanec, who helped me modify it for this play.

"Age of majority" in healthcare decision-making has been a hotly debated policy issue in many jurisdictions. In this regard, a well-known feminist ethicist asked me to consider writing a play to explore "what if" an intellectually advanced adolescent did not want to undergo the treatment strategy that had been decided upon by his physicians and agreed to by his parents. Philip surfaces the complexities of children developing intellectually at different rates, and affording the dignity of self-determination in decisions affecting their health.

---

[29] V. Bergum, *A Child on Her Mind: The Experience of Becoming a Mother*, West Port, CT: Bergin & Garvey, 1997.
[30] J.A. Nisker, Rachel's ladders, or how societal situation determines reproductive therapy, *Human Reproduction*, 1996, 11(6), 1162–1167; J.A. Nisker, In quest of the perfect analogy for using in vitro fertilization patients as oocyte donors, *Women's Health Issues*, 1997, 7(4), 241–247.
[31] S. Rogers, F. Baylis, A.Lippman, J. MacMillan, B. Parish, and J. Nisker, Policy statement: Preconception arrangements, *Journal of Obstetrics and Gynaecology Canada*, 1997, 19, 393–399.
[32] J. Nisker, Introduction to A Child on Her Mind, in V. Bergum, J. Van Der Zalm (eds.), *Mother Life: Studies of Mothering Experience*, Edmonton, AB: Pedagon Publishing, 2007, pp. 358–363.

Orchids explores diverse views of the concept of "normal" and the relationship of genetic inquiry to pursuing its quest. *Orchids* suggests pause for consideration of the reflection persons living with "disabilities" will see in genetic technology's magic mirror, consideration of how "normal" persons will view disabled reflections, will view their own image, will view humanity. As indicated earlier in this Introduction, *Orchids* was completed in 1995, and is based on my personal experiences researching the technology for preimplantation genetic diagnosis as well as the concerns of feminist writers. Indeed, the plot of *Orchids* was based on real-life possibilities in our clinic in 1993, and was prescient of today's ever-increasing possibilities regarding pre-designed children. Although genetic research has provided important information regarding the understanding of many serious conditions and has afforded choices regarding health promotion for persons living with genetic-related conditions (as explored in *Sarah's Daughters*), genetic research also tempts a "geneticized"[33] view of humanity. *Orchids* promotes sensitivity for those different from the scientific "ideal" and warns we should not perceive or attempt to achieve perfection.

Sarah's Daughters (completed 2001) and *Orchids* were also used to assess the possibility of theatre as a health policy development tool. The results were published in the journal *Health Policy*[34] in 2006 and in *Social Science and Medicine*[35] in 2009. The research using Orchids was funded by the Canadian Institutes of Health Research (CIHR) and Health Canada. The research using *Sarah's Daughters* was funded by Genome Canada and the Ontario Genomics Institute. More than 2,000 people saw performances of these plays as part of the research projects, and many more saw the plays in non-research productions. Post-performance theatre audience discussions and focus groups were taped and transcribed, and the transcripts underwent rigorous qualitative analysis.[36] The research indicated that theatre audience members were engaged both emotionally and cognitively in complex health policy issues and were able to offer informed opinions. This capacity of theatre stems from the ability of the director and actors to convey to the

---

[33] A. Lippman, The politics of health: Geneticization v. health promotion, in S. Sherwin and W. Mitchinson (eds.), *The Politics of Women's Health: Exploring Agency and Autonomy*, Philadelphia, PA: Temple University Press, 1988, pp. 64–82.

[34] J. Nisker, D. Martin, R. Bluhm, and A. Daar, Theatre as a public engagement tool for health-policy development, *Health Policy*, 2006, 78 (2–3), 258–271.

[35] S. Cox, M. Kazubowski-Houston, and J. Nisker, Genetics on stage: Public engagement in health policy development on preimplantation genetic diagnosis, *Social Science & Medicine*, 2009, 68(8), 1472–1480.

[36] A. Strauss and J. Corbin, *Basics of Qualitative Research*, Thousands Oaks, CA: Sage Publications, 1998.

audience the experiences and knowledge of both the persons interviewed for the script and the members of the communities who commented at script readings. When we hold post-performance audience discussions with the actors, audience members share their insights and receive further insight from each other, promoting multidirectional learning from the initial script development interviews, through the theatre audience discussions, and even perhaps to health policy makers.

I am committed to theatre as an essential tool for returning humanity to health ethics deliberation and health policy formation because I believe theatre can "help compassion happen."[37] Plays that promote compassion for the individual also promote compassion for the community. I hope you will find these plays useful for yourselves and your communities when considering health ethics issues and forwarding on health policies that insist on humanity in health promotion and care for everyone.

---

[37] J.A. Nisker, Orchids: Not necessarily a gospel, in J. Murray (ed.), *Mappa Mundi: Mapping Culture/Mapping the World*, Windsor, ON: University of Windsor Press, 2001, pp. 61–109.

Acknowledgements

This book was made possible through a University of Western Ontario Faculty Scholar Award for innovation. As this award was in recognition of my use of theatre as a public engagement tool for health policy development, I felt it appropriate to use the award to encourage others to write plays to bring issues of health policy to the public. The plays in the book have previously been published in whole or in part, and each publisher will be acknowledged separately with each play.

I would like to thank Mariko Obokata for her editorial assistance.

About the Author

Jeff Nisker is Coordinator of Health Ethics and Humanities, and Professor of Obstetrics-Gynaecology, at the Schulich School of Medicine & Dentistry, Western University. He has written or co-written more than 150 research articles and book chapters in the basic, clinical, and social sciences, and has edited or co-edited four books. Jeff has also written nine plays to encourage compassion in health promotion and care. His plays have been performed throughout Canada, in the United States, the United Kingdom, Australia, and South Africa. Jeff is the international member on the Board of Directors of the Center for Literature and Medicine (United States), has served on the editorial boards of the Journal of Medical Humanities and Ars Medica, and was Editor-in-Chief of the Journal of Obstetrics and Gynaecology Canada.

Jeff was co-chair of Health Canada's Advisory Committee on Reproductive and Genetic Technology and served on the Executive of the Canadian Bioethics Society. He has chaired and served on many national committees, including the Canadian Institutes of Health Research (CIHR) Standing Committee on Ethics, the National Council of Ethics in Human Research, the Society of Obstetricians and Gynaecologists of Canada Ethics Committee, and the Royal College of Physicians and Surgeons Ethics and Equity and Public Policy Committees. Jeff has received CIHR and Genome Canada grants to investigate the use of theatre for public engagement in health policy development; the understandings of patients, clinicians, and the general public in regard to genetic technology; and the effects of plasticizers on pregnant women.

Jeff has received many research and teaching awards. He was awarded the Society of Obstetricians and Gynaecologists of Canada President's Award for the most significant contribution to obstetrics and gynaecology in Canada. In 2008, Jeff won a Faculty Scholar Award for innovation in research and education that has enabled him to complete the new plays included in this book. Jeff was chosen by the Canadian Broadcasting Corporation's Peter Gzowski as one of the 13 "Best Minds of Our Time."

Calcedonies

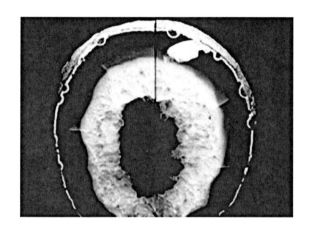

To the woman I call Ruth and to Catherine Frazee

Characters

Ruth, a woman in her late thirties or early forties.
Friend, a man the same age as Ruth.

Scene 1

To stage left is a small table on which sits a large mid-1990s Apple computer in classic translucent green. Large calcedony bookends sit prominently on the table, one on each side of the computer. Also on the table is a calcedony paperweight. Further to stage left is a narrow lectern facing away from audience. At stage right is a hospital bed, head cranked to 75° facing the audience. The bed is covered in white sheets and a hospital-blue blanket. Three IV bags are suspended from two "T-poles" inserted into the head of the bed. A hospital television set is suspended from a similar pole on the right side of the bed. A semicircle of simple straight-back chairs perimeters the stage, open to the audience. A large picture of the calcedony bookends is suspended stage back behind the chairs. During the memorial service scenes, coloured lights are projected onto this image to mimic cathedral-like hues.

Friend sits in the first chair of the semicircle stage front and right, head bowed, eyes open. Friend wears a black sport jacket over a black T-shirt and tan slacks. Lights for group home up on stage. Spot on Ruth as she zooms onto stage in her power wheelchair. From the power chair's right armrest extends a chin-operated joystick. Ruth charges across stage front and pirouettes. Ruth gets out of chair and walks to desk (with assistance if required). Ruth wears a peasant dress popular in the late 1960s and early 1970s. Ruth has a large colourfully patched and fringed handbag of that time, which she either carries on her shoulder or on her chair. A large agate pendant hangs from her neck on a black leather strap.

Ruth: Calcedonies are rocks,

Crusty-surfaced rocks

That open to amethyst, agate, onyx, chrysoprase

And become jewellery, paperweights, bookends,

For into each one's core,

Millennia have poured alloyed amazement.

Depending on their community,

They endow their bearers with wisdom,

Courage,

Healing powers.

Spiritual powers.

Each calcedony is unique,

Wonderfully one of a kind.

Friends used to give me calcedonies as gifts.

Because I love them.

Calcedonies and them.

Like this paperweight

[Lifts paperweight and places it back on desk]

And this agate

[Lifts pendant from neck]

My favourite calcedonies are my bookends.

[Lifts one in each hand, does three arm curls, feigns fatigue, returns them]

My bookends now bookend my computer,

Cause my books ended.

Seventeen years without turning a page.

My computer waits patiently for me

To press its power button.

And I will one day.

Then these arcs on my bookends will become my rainbow.

And my computer will fly me over my rainbow

To a better-than-emerald place,

From which I will never return.

[Walks (with assistance if required) to the picture of bookends. Indicates bookends in poster stage back, using the laser pointer, as if delivering a lecture.]

Don't my bookends look like a brain

On a TV doctor's MRI screen?

The "cerebral cortex."

The fluid-filled "ventricles."

Their brain resemblance reminds me

That I have a neurological condition.

[Walking to power chair]

Not that I need bookends to remind me

That my brain no longer speaks to my muscles,

Any of my muscles.

Except those that open my eyes,

Move my eyeballs,

Breathe me,

And, most important, move my jaw.

My other muscles are useless.

So you're probably wondering how I can walk around

like this?

Fine, I'll sit down if it's bothering you.

[Ruth sits in power chair and positions her chin on joystick.]

My brain still works.

Exceptionally well actually,

As I'm sure you've already noticed.

Even my doctors think my brain works exceptionally well.

But as they see the rest of my body as so un-well,

It's easy for them to see my brain as exceptional.

I guess it's better to have a well brain than a well body.

I mean if you had to choose one or the other.

At least I think so.

[Quickly moves chair to other side of stage]

I know you can't wait to hear more about my amazing

brain muscles,

But first I must tell you about my amazing jaw muscles.

My jaw muscles allow me to speak,

Albeit very quietly,

And seldom heard.

They open my mouth so I can eat,

Although an attendant at the group home

Has to shovel the food in.

And most important,

My jaw muscles work this joystick on my chair,

The magic wand that propels me to the joy I have left.

Like dancing.

[Ruth dances around stage in power chair in graceful arcs to "Unchained Melody," Righteous Brothers' version, then to Michael Jackson's "Billie Jean." Ruth "moonwalks" the chair backward to a wing, then races it across the stage front, turns to face audience.]

Not bad, eh?

Now where was I?

Each morning I patiently wait to be cleaned up,

Bum loaded into chair,

Chin placed on joystick,

Head strapped down.

But when the patient wait is finally over,

Which might be noon,

My joystick frees me.

At least to dash around the group home:

TV room, dining room, back to bedroom.

[Stands and walks across stage to hospital bed]

When I'm in hospital,

And recovered enough from what got me here,

Sometimes someone has the time

To get me into my chair.

Then I really have fun.

[Walks back to chair facing audience and sits in it with chin on joystick and hands on imaginary steering wheel]

I bomb down the halls at full throttle,

Pick up some serious speed,

Pick off a doctor or two.

I've made a blood sport of it.

When I spot a doctor down the hall,

I stop my chair.

Slowly move my jaw left or right,

Turning my chair's front wheels

To aim at the doctor's white coat,

As if it was a matador's red cape.

My left foot stamps the sand of the bullring.

[Uses left hand for stomping motion]

Then I push my jaw as forward as possible,

Charging at the matadoctor like a ferocious bull.

Doctors never notice me until I'm almost on them

Because patients are invisible to doctors.

But when they see me bearing down upon them,

With no intention of swerving from my bloody course,

Surprise then terror grips their eyes,

And they plaster themselves against the nearest wall,

Or dodge into a patient's room.

I love scaring the shit out of doctors.

It's the most fun I ever have.

And I really do scare the shit out of some doctors.

My sense of smell still works, you know.

And I always take a quick sniff as I speed by.

Of course I'm used to the smell of shit,

Steeping in it as I do

While patiently waiting for someone to clean me up.

Anyway, unlike matadors,

Matadoctors never beckon me to another charge.

In fact they usually flee next time they see me.

But just like matadors kill bulls,

The matadoctors will kill me in the end.

The crowd may even cheer.

[Ruth sits in chair, places her chin on joystick and freezes.]

Scene 2

[Lights fade to memorial service with spot on Friend again. Friend slowly lifts head.]

Friend: I sit amidst a "Circle of Friends,"

     Eight women,

     None who know me.

     "It will be a simple service,"

     I was told on the phone.

     I said I had "another commitment,"

     "A son's soccer practice,"

     And apologized.

     "You might say a few words."

     I apologized again.

     "Only if you're so moved."

     Rainbows pour from the simple windows,

     Melting their art on the silent circle.

     All eyes are open,

     Staring downward.

     All hearts are open,

     Embracing her life;

     Except my heart,

     Fixed in the formaldehyde of her death.

23

Scene 3

[Lights up for hospital room. Ruth stands and walks to stage front.]

Ruth: Let me tell you more about my body.

I could be burned at the stake like Joan of Arc,

And feel no pain.

At least until my chin caught fire.

The no-pain thing amazes medical students.

They come to practise neurological exams on me all the time I'm in,

Which always includes the infamous pinprick test.

You don't know what the pinprick test is?

Little pricks... prick your skin... with little pins... to determine

Which areas of skin are still connected to your brain.

I refer to all medical students as "little pricks,"

Having no insight into their true prick size.

And of course there're more women in medical school

Than when I first became a voodoo doll.

If a medical student acts like an arrogant prick,

I mess him up a bit.

Like by shrieking in pain when they prick me,

Or screaming "Fuck!"

24

It's a hoot watching them flinch,

Apologizing profusely.

One little prick actually pricked himself.

[Sits on bed]

So why am I in hospital getting pricked?

I get pressure sores

"Down there"

Because we who can't feel pressure

"Down there"

Can't shift the weight off our butts

The way you who can feel your butts

Do all the time without realizing it.

They sometimes call these things bedsores,

Though the bed doesn't get sore.

And if a bedsore gets infected,

We get admitted to hospital

For IV antibiotics.

I once made a nurse show me

What my infected bedsore looked like.

She had to use two mirrors

To show me a dollar-size circle of black, red, and yellow

crud.

Sort of an angry archery target.

One look was enough, thank you very much.

[Ruth sits back in chair and moves along stage front with occasional loops, flourishes and other waltz-like moves, and she stops stage centre.]

Before I went from "able-bodied" to chin-bodied,

From free spirit to —

Well, I'm still a free spirit,

But could easily be much freer

If I could just fucking get my joystick connected to my

computer.

Sorry about that.

I was a sculptor:

Amazed each day by the beauty

Glazes baked on my clay,

And coloured enamel bits melted on my carved copper.

I formed a special relationship with my copper kiln.

He was my partner in creating jewellery.

Yes, my kiln is a "he."

His name is Fred.

And he was so much my partner in creation

That the sign on my studio read "Ruth and Fred."

When I was moved into my first chronic care "facility,"

I gave away my furniture, clothes, kitchen things,

Even my books,

But I couldn't give Fred away.

So I asked a friend to keep him for me in her garage.

He might still be there.

I know that Fred will never help me create again.

But I will create again.

Through poetry.

[In voice from The Six Million Dollar Man]

"We have the technology,"

[Ruth walks over to her computer and smiles.]

It's an Apple.

[Looks fondly at computer]

Apple developed disability-friendly software years ago.

So I cashed in my life savings to buy this beauty.

[Caresses computer]

My chin will operate it through my joystick

The way your hand uses a mouse.

Only I won't need a mouse pad.

The software platform will be my rocket-launching pad,

And I will blast off from this world of exclusion,

And I will never "re-enter."

It has voice-activated software,

Called "Dragon."

Dragon will allow me to communicate with people

And to write the poems

I have collected in my heart for so many years.

I will speak a line,

See the words appear on the screen,

Spend all day gently massaging the words

As they gently massage me.

But a bio-med-i-cal engineer is required

To calibrate my jaw with the computer program

That will interface my face with my computer's face.

I've been on the waiting list for over a year now.

And was told it could be another two-year wait.

Because there're only two bio-med-i-cal engineers in our
"Region"

Who can connect the umbilical cords of people "like me."

And no more can be hired.

Because of the fucking funding cutbacks.

Sorry again.

So I wait.

I patiently wait.

Scene 4

[Ruth stands, exits stage right, and returns quickly with a hospital gurney. Two IV poles are attached to the head of the gurney, and three plastic IV bags hang from the poles, their IV tubing pinned to the stretcher under the white sheet. Ruth pushes the stretcher to stage front centre and orients it parallel to stage front. Ruth then lies on the stretcher and covers herself with the white sheet. Once Ruth covers herself with the sheet, Friend walks to stage centre behind the stretcher and faces the audience. The lights come down on them.]

Friend: The patient's face seems familiar to me,

As the Clinical Fellow rapidly presents

The patient's history and clinical findings.

[Rapidly]

A three-centimetre infected bed sore, ulcerating skin of

vulva,

Just south and to left of vagina.

Came in unconscious through ER three nights ago.

Total body sepsis from spread of infection from bedsore.

Triple antibiotic therapy.

Still out of it.

Nothing more we can do for bed sore,

Or for her for that matter.

Quadriplegic.

[Pause]

Quadriplegic.

I knew I've seen this woman before.

In fact I've seen her several times over the years,

Racing down our hospital's halls in her electric wheelchair.

I remember once she lost control of her chair

And almost plowed me over.

I remind the Clinical Fellow to always treat my patients as if

they're fully awake.

He quips, "We're not in the operating room,"

An attempt at a joke as I am well known (and derided)

For insisting my anesthetized patients always be treated as if

they are awake.

I have insisted this ever since I was a Clinical Fellow,

And a large woman had written on her abdomen prior to

surgery

"No fat jokes please," in indelible ink.

The Clinical Fellow urges, "She really can't hear us,"

Then shouts at her,

[Shouting]

"Do — you — know — where — you —are?"

Then claps his hands in front of her face.

31

[Claps loudly three times]

[Pauses with Friend staring at Ruth's eyes]

> I ask our patient's name.
>
> He replies, "Ruth ___."
>
>
> Hello Ruth,
>
> I'm sorry that you're not feeling well.

[Pause]

> Ruth, I need to examine the bedsore on your vulva.
>
> The Clinical Fellow gives me his "Don't you trust me"
>
> look

[Pause]

> You may not be able to give me your permission,
>
> But it is important that I examine your bedsore.
>
>
> The nurse helps me position the white sheet below
>
> Ruth's knees.
>
> We gently lift the emaciated calf muscles
>
> Upward and outward to the "frog leg" position.
>
> I part the white curtains
>
> To the infected ulceration.
>
> I say to myself, "I hope the antibiotics can ameliorate this,

I don't think surgery is the answer."

I close the curtains.

I say to Ruth, what I'm sure she has heard so many times

before,

"I'm sorry, but there's nothing more we can do."

Then I pull the chart from the Clinical

Fellow's hands.

He is taken aback

Because I've never done this before.

He urges, "They must be ready to start our case in the

OR."

I flip back the pages to the very beginning.

[Pause]

Ruth's date of birth and mine are identical:

Same year, same month, same day.

My eyes rivet the hundreds of haunting pages.

Scene 5

[Ruth gets out of gurney and lies on hospital bed (60° up) facing audience. Friend pushes gurney into wing, returns to his chair and sits.]

Ruth: I have another bedsore,

And this one got infected,

Really infected.

And the infection spread through my body so quickly

That by the time the ambulance got me to

Emerg —

[Friend stands and hesitantly takes a few steps towards Ruth.]

I'll have to tell you about that later

Because some strange doctor has just come into my room.

[Friend keeps looking over shoulder back at the door as he walks even more hesitantly toward Ruth.]

I think he's in the wrong room.

That happens sometimes.

His first words to me are,

[Friend continues walking hesitantly toward Ruth.]

Friend: I am no longer your physician.

Ruth: Like God talking to Moses in The Ten Commandments.

So I carefully choose my first words to him.

Who the fuck are you?

But as I'm still weak from infection

"Fuck" comes out quieter than usual,

So he's not sure he heard me right.

Or can't believe he heard me right.

[Friend looks like he wants to leave, but he takes a chair, places it close to head of bed, sits on chair, and brings his ear close to Ruth's lips.]

Ruth: *[Loud]*

Who-the-fuck-are-you?

[Friend jolts back]

Friend: I'm sorry, I'm Doctor _____.

Ruth: Let's leave out his name to protect the guilty.

Friend: May I speak with you for a few minutes?

Ruth: Well Doc, you're really lucky

I just happen to have some free time in my crowded social

calendar

Because my Pilates class was cancelled.

Friend: *[Sheepishly]*

I want to apologize to you.

Ruth: You should, Doc,

It's late and I need my beauty sleep

If I'm ever going to hump a pole again.

[Friend looks stunned, hesitates, then plods onward.]

Friend: I'm apologizing for watching the colours of your TV set

           Reflect on your face while you were sleeping last night.

Ruth: Doc, if you were that interested in what was on TV,

           You could've turned the TV around to watch it.

[Friend looks stunned.]

           No sense of humour,

           No doctors have a sense of humour.

           But get this, after watching my face for a bit,

           He, and these are his exact words,

Friend: Felt like a voyeur

Ruth: So he decided to leave.

           But before he left, he shut off the TV,

           And separated its neckset arms from my ears.

Friend: To let you sleep more peacefully.

Ruth: But when he stepped out of my room,

Friend: I froze in a shower of stupidity

Ruth: Because he realized that if I woke up

Friend: You wouldn't be able to turn the TV back on,

Ruth: Nor press the button to call a nurse to turn it back on.

Friend: You'd just stare at the dark screen

Because of my—

Ruth & Friend:

Misplaced assistance.

Ruth: I like "stupidity" better.

Friend: So I returned and moved the TV back to where I thought it was,

Turned it back on to the same channel, I hope,

And placed the audio pieces back in your ears."

Ruth: Very strange doctor.

Friend: I also want to apologize

For examining you last week when you were unconscious.

[Pause]

Without your permission.

Ruth: Whoa.

Really, Doc.

And exactly what part of me

Did you examine without my permission?

Friend: I examined the bedsore on your vulva.

Ruth: *[Pause]*

O…K…

I really thought doctors couldn't say anything to throw me off anymore.

So of course I make him explain in great detail what a "VULVA" is,

Insisting on all the anatomical and functional details.

[To Friend]

And what exactly did you do to my "VULVA" Doc?

Let me summarize:

He looked at my crotch,

And, yes, he touched my crotch.

I clearly must've been out of it

Because that's the sort of thing a gal remembers,

Even if she can't feel her VULVA.

Friend: I'm glad you don't remember me.

I don't want any vestige of doctor–patient relationship to exist.

Ruth: Vestige?

Friend: Because I want to ask your permission to visit you as a friend.

You're free to say no,

Or, if you say yes now,

You can change your mind at any time later.

Ruth: He's asking my permission in such a formal way,

That I'm surprised he doesn't shove a consent form in my face,

And put a pen in my hand to sign it.

Not that he wouldn't have, if I could have.

He says he's written a note on my chart

Dissolving our physician–patient relationship,

And asked a colleague to see me in follow-up.

So why do you want to be my friend, Doc?

If you stay my doctor

You can bill the system for visiting me.

Even bill double for a Sunday night like tonight.

Even if you don't look at my VULVA anymore.

Although I must have one hell of a VULVA.

[Friend tries to speak but freezes with stunned look again.]

Ruth: Now why exactly did you want to be my friend instead of my doctor?

Friend: We have identical dates of birth.

Ruth: What?

Friend: We were born the same year, same month, same day.

Ruth: Born same day.

This is getting

[Sings Twilight Zone tune]

Don't tell me that in addition to looking at my VULVA

You actually looked at my chart.

Only nurses and medical students ever look at a patient's

chart.

[To audience]

Being exactly the same age has connected him with me

in some way.

Probably in a there-but-for-the-grace-of-God-go-I way.

[Friend turns and begins to walk out but stops.]

Friend: Ruth, the arms of the TV's audioset in your ears last night

Made it look like you were wearing a stethoscope,

Listening to the TV's heartbeat.

[Friend turns again to leave.]

Ruth: *[In a Rocky Balboa voice]*

> Yo, Doc,
>
> If you're not too busy,
>
> Drop in after work tomorrow.

*[To audience]*Better than boredom.

Friend: I'd love to, but tomorrow is Monday.

Ruth: *Monday, no kidding, Doc?*

> Quads do know the days of the week.

[Friend looks stunned again.]

Friend: On Monday nights, I do an elective for our medical students.

Ruth: An elective?

Friend: It means that the students are not required to attend.

Ruth: Then why would they?

Friend: I guess they come because they like what we discuss.

Ruth: And what about those who don't come?

Friend: Most of the guys stay home and watch

> Monday Night Football. Sorry, I really have to go.

[Friend quickly leaves.]

Scene 6

[Spot on Ruth as she gets into chair and wheels to beside back-facing lectern and faces audience. Second spot on Friend as he enters and hurries toward lectern but encounters Ruth on the way.]

Ruth: He hurries into the hospital's lecture theatre

      Seconds before he's scheduled to begin.

      He sees me right away.

      He has no choice,

      As my chair is right in front of the front doors.

      I have no choice,

      As wheelchairs can only enter at the front,

      And then there are steps.

      I can tell he wants to start his class,

      But he just keeps staring at me,

      Probably wondering how I got a doctor to write the order

      For me to leave the ward.

      (No order of course was ever written)

      And how I knew where the lecture theatre was.

      (I've been displayed here several times over the years)

      He forces his stare away from me

      To smile at the hundred or so medical students behind me,

      Who are also trying not to stare at me.

      But stare anyway,

Looking for clues to what I have:

Half-filled piss bag beside my chair's left wheel,

No movement of limbs,

Head supported front and back.

Obviously something neuromuscular.

Car accident quads aren't interesting enough

To be displayed in large lecture hall.

His feet come even closer to mine,

So he's sure I can see him.

He thanks me for coming and tells me

Friend: You're looking very well tonight.

Ruth: Give me a break.

          Then he quickly asks my permission

          To introduce me to the students

Friend: Not as a patient here but as your friend.

Ruth: He wants my permission again.

          Why not introduce me as someone born the identical day as
          you?

[Friend starts to speak but stops.]

          Hey Doc, what do you think of my slippers?

          He looks down at my furry bear paw slippers,

Complete with black felt claws.

He's just about to tell me how much he likes my slippers

When I interrupt again with, "I've had these for years."

[Friend opens mouth and freezes again.]

He's trying to determine whether I'm making a joke

(Because slippers don't wear out when you don't walk

on them),

Or am I innocently applauding the staff for not losing them

(Me, innocent?),

Or am I trying to throw him off

His carefully thought-out introduction to tonight's

"exploration"?

Finally he forces his jaw to work

And fumblingly welcomes the students and introduces the

topic.

He then smiles and takes a deep breath:

Friend: We have a guest with us tonight,

My friend, Ruth.

Scene 7

[Ruth gets onto the bed and covers herself.]

Ruth: Now that I've made my way back to my room,

Been lifted back into bed,

Piss bag changed,

Teeth brushed,

TV channel turned to the one I've calculated

To have the fewest bad shows till I fall asleep,

Let me tell you what the medical students got tonight.

Seven student "volunteers" came to the front

And took turns reading stanzas of two poems by Rilke.

I knew the one about the panther

Pacing the perimeter of its cage,

Paralyzed by the bars.

Then the students watched part of a film

About a man in Victorian England,

Who had these huge lumps on his body,

And had to hide or be taunted.

Scene 8

Friend: When I walked into the meeting room,

I was again asked to "Share a few words."

I repeated I could not.

"Only if you want to."

I apologized again.

"Only when you're ready to."

I knew I never would be ready to,

Reeking of remorse about her life,

Guilt about her death.

[Looks across at semicircle of chairs]

The woman who met me at the door lifts her eyes,

And tells a warm anecdote about "our Friend."

She finishes too soon for me.

The ensuing silence consumes me.

I feel all eyes upon me

Finally another woman lifts her eyes,

And speaks about "our Friend's" great sense of humour.

All smile,

[Pause]

Except me.

Scene 9

[Ruth in peasant dress sits in her chair and wheels to beside back-facing lectern and faces audience.]

Ruth: This time he runs in

With a whole three minutes to spare.

Of course, I sit in the same place.

Of course, he gives me the same stunned look,

Friend: I'm sorry you're back in hospital.

Ruth: I'm not back in hospital.

A van that moves us disableds

Out of our storage facilities and back in again

Got me here.

Friend: I'm glad you're not ill again.

Ruth: Then he quickly welcomes the students before I can throw him off,

And finishes with

Friend: Our friend, Ruth, has joined us again.

Ruth: This Monday Night's not as powerful.

Just one very long one-woman Victorian play

About mental illness.

The strange doc-who-wants-to-be-my-friend

Told the students he adapted it from a short story

With "permission of the estate of the author."

I did like the way the play showed

How women can be confined by the times in which they

live,

And by the medical profession.

I also liked the medical student actor.

She didn't miss one line

Of those thousands and thousands of lines.

I'll bet she'll remember every line of every medical

textbook she reads.

She also seemed very sensitive.

I want her to be my doctor on both counts.

When the "exploration" is over,

A bunch of students surround me,

Asking how I'm feeling,

How I liked the play,

What I thought of their buddy's memorization skill.

Out of the corner of my eye I see my strange doctor,

Grinning like a Cheshire cat.

After all the students are gone,

He walks over, still smiling,

And asks if he can "accompany me" to the van.

I rapidly lead onward.

He stupidly walks behind my chair

As if he's pushing it.

When we come to the closed doors

Separating the lecture halls from the rest of the hospital,

He dashes round my chair,

And bows as he opens the doors for me.

So gal<u>o</u>nt.

[Speeds wheelchair across front side of stage]

I speed down the hall to the elevators.

He catches up puffing, blushing, apologizing.

Eventually it dawns on him to press the down button.

He smiles.

The elevator comes quickly as "Visiting hours are now over."

I pirouette my chair and quickly back in.

He presses G,

Then proceeds to tell about his claustrophobia

Since a teenager because of a recurring dream.

Just as the elevator doors open to the ground floor,

[Speeds wheelchair to centre stage]

I make a beeline for the front doors

Even though I know the automatic doors don't work after nine.

He catches up and smiles.

I tell him, I would like to wait outside,

It's a beautiful evening after all.

He proudly presses the door's "ALARM WILL

SOUND" lever-bar,

Telling me, It's okay, the alarm won't sound,

I always use this door at night to quickly get to my car.

[Speeds wheelchair to opposite side of stage]

I dash out, turn left, and stop before the sign

Prohibiting smoking near the doors.

My strange-doctor friend catches up

And asks my "permission" to wait with me.

I tell him, The van's usually late,

May not be here for an hour.

Friend: I would still like to wait with you if that's okay,

It's a beautiful evening after all.

Ruth: Okay Doc, then make yourself useful,

Fetch me a cig from the sack behind my chair.

50

Friend: You smoke?

Ruth: Of course not, smoking would be bad for my health.

He tries not to glance at the no smoking sign.

I don't tell him that I always smoke in front of this sign,

Just to see if any security guard has the rocks

To make me move further from the door.

They never do.

Afraid of me for some reason.

Maybe they think they'll catch what I got.

My cigs, please.

[Friend hesitantly walks to back of chair and very gingerly places his hand in sack.]

He's carefully feeling around in my sack,

Probably embarrassed to have his hand in a woman's purse,

Afraid of what he might touch.

[Friend finally pulls out the pack of Marlboros and holds it in front of Ruth's face.]

Friend: I found them.

Ruth: Now take a cig out of the pack.

[Friend slowly draws cigarette out of pack.]

He's drawing it out of the pack

As if it's a nuclear rod.

Now into my mouth, please.

Come on, I promise not to tell anyone that you're

hastening my death.

He's a blushing iceberg,

But I'm getting really pissed off.

You'd be pissed off too if a cig was taunting you

Mere inches from your mouth.

Just put the fucking thing in my mouth!

Friend: Fine.

[Shoves cigarette deep into Ruth's mouth]

Ruth: *[choking]*

Take it out.

Friend: Sorry, sorry, sorry, sorry—.

Ruth: Just put it back in!

But just a little way this time.

[Friend very gently places the cigarette at the edge of Ruth's lips. Ruth tightly clamps on to cigarette, rotating her lips to move it further into her mouth.]

Friend: In okay?

Ruth: Would I be working my mouth like a camel if it's IN OKAY?

Friend: Sorry.

[Gently pushes cigarette in further]

Ruth: He stands there like a dolt

          Staring at my cig,

          I sit here like a patient woman,

          Staring at his stupid face.

          You don't expect me just to suck on it

          Like a fucking candy cigarette?

Friend: I'm sorry. Do you have any matches in your purse?

Ruth: *[Glaring at Friend]*

          He cautiously excavates my purse again

          While I'm dying here.

[Friend embarrassed with hand in purse. Then raises matches high in victory, proud of himself, and then holds them in front of Ruth's face.]

Friend: Do you want me to light your cigarette for you?

Ruth: I'm ready to kill him but instead say,

[In Billy Crystal's Fernando Lamas's voice]

          That would be M-A-H-V-E-L-O-U-S,

          That is, if you think you can light it without burning my face.

          But the joke's on me.

          He fumbles with the matches like he's never lit one before.

          He scratches and scratches,

          Finally a flame,

53

But it goes out before it reaches my cig.

Because his hands are shaking like he has a neurological

problem himself.

I'm glad he's never going to operate on me.

I wish I could steady his hands in mine like in the movies.

[Next match gets to cigarette and Ruth frantically puffs.]

The fucking flame went out.

Friend: Okay, okay.

[Scratches match after match and puts flame to cigarette]

Ruth: *[Puffs and puffs then]*

Ahh ... Ahh ... Ahh.

Friend: You look like a movie gangster,

With the cigarette in the corner of your mouth like that.

[Ruth cradles cigarette in corner of mouth. Ignores him.]

Friend: *[In movie gangster voice]*

Tell me everything.

Ruth: I think he's trying to make a gangster movie joke,

I go with it though.

I've committed no crimes I know of.

Then instead of telling him "everything" about me,

54

I tell him "everything" about his healthcare system,

And what he can do with it.

I love how he flinches in pain

Each time I skewer his profession,

Which he apparently loves,

And definitely has endless excuses for.

Like,

Friend: We've less than half the doctors per citizen of any developed

country,

Ruth: Like,

Friend: We do the best we can under hospital funding cutbacks,

Ruth: Like

Friend: Don't blame the physicians

Blame the politicians,

And the citizens who voted them in

For personal income tax cuts.

Ruth: All the while he tries not to stare at the bobbing ash of my cig.

Or at the ash falling on my shawl.

I know he wants to brush the ash off

But he's afraid to touch me.

[Friend timidly brushes air above shawl.]

Now he's worrying the cig's getting too short

And my lips will burn.

Friend: Can I take it out?

Ruth: Sure if it's making you nervous,

But you're wasting good tobacco.

[Friend gently removes the butt and looks for a place to dump it.]

Light me another thank-you-very-much.

[Friend searches purse again, then remembers Marlboros are on the ground where he dropped them.]

I usually have just one cig in the evening.

But it's such a riot watching this doctor struggle

That I keep asking him to light me cig after cig.

He tries not to look relieved when the van arrives.

I try not to look disappointed,

But I was hoping the driver forgot about me.

That happens you know.

Tonight's driver,

A burly guy about our age,

Walks round to our side of the van.

He smiles as he swings open the barn doors,

And presses the button that lowers the elevator platform.

I gun my chair forward onto the platform,

Thanks for the drags, Doc.

And am hauled up and into the van

As there's no room to turn my chair,

I stare out the window on the opposite side

At a vacant bus shelter and a yellowish street light.

I hear the ratcheting down of my chair to the van's floor,

Then the metallic thud of the closed doors.

The driver walks past the window.

His weight enters the van.

The motor rumbles on,

The bus shelter and street light move left and are gone.

Suddenly I see my strange-doctor friend running beside the window,

Frantically waving goodbye with both hands,

And mouthing like an orangutan,

T-H-A-N-K Y-O-U F-O-R C-O-M-I-N-G

He's going to get hit by a car.

He keeps this up for a while,

But finally disappears left.

Probably collapsed on the street.

Scene 10

[Ruth wheels to centre stage front.]

Ruth: I'm back in hospital for some plumbing problems.

Nothing serious.

I saw my strange-doctor-supposed-friend today

While I was bombing down the halls on his floor.

Too bad he saw me coming,

And jumped out of the way,

Or I would have flattened him good.

With all his "I want to be friends" bullshit,

He never visited me at the group home.

Not once in six months.

And it's so close to the hospital.

Anyway after he peeled himself off the wall,

He asked my room number so he could visit me later,

And dashed off.

Scene 11

[Friend walks to centre stage front, stands beside Ruth, and speaks to the audience.]

Friend: I saw Ruth while I was waiting for an elevator.

   She was hurrying over to say hello,

   But lost control of her wheelchair,

   And almost crashed into me.

   I told her how glad I was to see her,

   But she misunderstood and said,

   You're glad I'm back in this —

[Pause]

   Place.

   She used an adjective before "place"

   Because she doesn't like hospitals.

   I was late for a meeting so couldn't talk to her,

   But I'll try to see her after work.

Scene 12

[Ruth gets into bed.]

Ruth: All patients learn to be patient.

That's why we're called "patients."

We have no choice but to be patient patients,

Except for some rich patients,

Who are "connected."

And patient patients are invisible while they wait:

Invisible to doctors obviously,

But also to nurses and receptionists.

Family members also learn to be patient.

And they don't get a dime for waiting room time,

Or transportation time,

Or help at home time.

But I am "no longer patient."

I need my joystick connected to my computer.

Now.

I've waited almost three years,

And can't fucking wait any longer.

There are things I want to learn,

Places I want to see,

Words I need to write.

And no doctor thought I'd live this long.

Scene 13

[Ruth is sitting up in hospital bed. Friend rushes over and mimes caring and concern gestures while Ruth speaks.]

Ruth: *[To audience]*

He rushes into my room after six.

Starts with his usual greeting, caring, concern for my health.

But, like all doctors, he's already got one foot out the door.

Doesn't even have time to draw the curtain around my bed.

After less than a minute of the bullshit he looks at his feet,

As he always does just before he starts apologizing for

having to leave,

Then, as usual, he asks me

Friend: Is there anything you need

Ruth: I always just stare.

He always just leaves.

But this time his feet don't move.

Friend: Since you're back in hospital and looking so well

Ruth: *[To audience]*

Something's coming.

Probably wants some students to see me or something.

Friend: Would you give me permission to bring my children in to

meet you?

Ruth: *[To audience]*

> Well, well, well.
>
> And he hasn't surprised me for a while.

Friend: It would only be for a few minutes.

> But I'd like you to say a few words to them.
>
> But only if you want to.
>
> And only if you're feeling well enough to.
>
> Please feel free to say no.

Ruth: Does this nutbar think I could possibly say,

> No, I'd rather not meet your kids?
>
> "Permission" to bring in your kids,
>
> Give me a break.
>
> So of course I say

[To Friend]

> I'm dying to meet your kids,

Friend: Thank you, I'll bring them to your room in an hour or so.

[Turns and starts leaving]

Ruth: Wait a second,

> Let's meet in my favourite part of the hospital.

Friend: *[Hesitantly]*

Favourite part?

Ruth: You know where,

Friend: *[Hesitates again]*

I do?

Ruth: Outside the front doors,

Friend: Well, I don't —ah—

Ruth: It's a beautiful evening after all.

Friend: I'm not sure it's a —

Ruth: I promise not to smoke in front of your kids,

Friend: Thank you.

[Turns and starts to leave]

Ruth: But only if you tell me about your recurring dream.

Friend: Recurring dream?

Ruth: The one that makes you claustrophobic in elevators.

Friend: I can't.

Ruth: Then I might just ask you in front of your kids

If you would join me in another cigarette.

Marlboros are your favourites aren't they, Macho Man?

Friend: I'd rather not talk about my dream.

Ruth: You'd rather not talk about anything having to do with you.

          But I really want to know about your dream.

          Maybe I can help you get over your claustrophobia.

Friend: You'll think I'm ridiculous.

Ruth: Not to worry.

          I already find you ridiculous.

          Now put your ass in that chair,

          Pretend it's a couch,

          And tell me your dream.

[Friend sits tentatively and looks down.]

Friend: There's a tumultuous lake.

Ruth: Very original.

[Friend gets up.]

Ruth: I'm sorry.

[Yawns]

          I promise not to interrupt again.

Friend: *[Sits]*

          We're standing on a pier,

          We, being the neighbours on my childhood block.

          A 14-year-old me

Stands between my mother and Mrs. Warner,

The beautiful woman who lives next door.

Mrs. Warner is holding the hand of her five-year-old son,

Jamie.

Suddenly a hard wave smashes into the pier

And sweeps Jamie into the roiling water.

He looks at me just before he's sucked down.

My mother grasps my arm and turns me toward her.

Her eyes beseech, "Don't."

I love my mother

But I'm the strongest swimmer on the street.

I dive in, but can't find Jamie.

I duck dive again and again.

I see a cave under the pier.

I swim in a ways and find Jamie.

He's very frightened.

I mouth, "Everything will be okay,"

Grasp his hand and turn to swim him out.

But there are two tunnels.

I choose one and swim Jamie down it,

But it gets narrower and narrower.

I have trouble turning us around.

I swim back as hard as I can.

I feel Jamie's body go limp.

I drag him with all that I have,

Running out of breath.

[Gasping]

Fighting panic with every stroke,

[Gasping]

And wake up gasping for air,

[Gasping]

Drenched in water.

Ruth: You mean sweat.

Friend: *[Pauses, still gasping]*

Ruth: Okay, we're making progress here.

Besides elevators what else gives your claustrophóbia?

Friend: Being buried in the sand by my kids.

Being buried in the sand is the worst.

Ruth: For me, too.

[Friend stares at Ruth then quickly leaves.]

Scene 14

Ruth: *[Gets out of bed and goes to front of stage]*

I wonder what he's told his kids about me.

Maybe she's like that guy in the Star Trek episode,

Where all that remains of him

Is his head mounted on a brainwave-operated wheelchair

After a radiation explosion.

I've seen that episode many times.

Seen all the Star Treks many times

Like every other series in syndication.

You know, I think that episode is called "The Menagerie."

Well the nurses do call this place "a zoo" when things get
crazy busy,

Which is most of the time.

So bring on the kids,

Let them see the most ferocious animal in this fucking zoo.

Scene 15

Friend: I pick up my sons,

Take them to "Wendy's Pick-up Window,"

Where they order grilled chicken with broccoli-cheddar

baked potatoes,

As trained to,

And head back to the hospital.

There is silence in the car except for chewing jaws.

My mind is immersed in the novel To Kill a Mockingbird,

The part where Atticus Finch sends his twelve-year-old son

Jem

To read to a seemingly unconscious woman.

Jem would rather be doing anything else during his summer

holidays

Than reading all afternoon to a woman who can't even hear him.

A nurse comes in now and then and sends Jem out for a few

minutes.

Over the weeks, Jem notices that the nurse comes in less

frequently,

Then not at all,

And that the woman gradually acknowledges him more and

more.

When the woman dies, Atticus explains to his son

That the woman had insisted on backing off the medicine

That took away her pain but made her sleepy

Because she wanted to fully experience life again before she died.

Atticus was teaching his son courage.

Scene 16

[Ruth sits in hospital bed. Friend sits beside her.]

Ruth: He's come alone to see me three nights in a row.

Three nights in a row is a new world's record,

And I guess his way of thanking me for permission to bring

his kids in.

They were very quiet.

I was very quiet.

That is until we started talking about movies.

I asked what their favourite movies are.

One said, The Great Escape,

Another, "The Bridge on the River Kwai.

The third said, Ghostbusters.

Tonight when my strange doctor friend asks before he leaves,

Friend: *[Friend stands and turns to leave]*

Is there anything you need?

Ruth: Instead of just staring,

I whisper, Hey, you born-the-identical-day-as-me,

Friend: Yes?

Ruth: I need my chair's joystick hooked up to my computer.

Friend: *[Laughing]*

I'm sorry but my experience with computers is confined

To helping my kids find Carmen Sandiego.

[Friend leaves but comes back in a few seconds and pulls up chair.]

Ruth: He draws the drapes around my bed.

Friend: I'm sorry. Tell me about —

[Blackout]

Scene 17

[Spot on Friend standing beside lectern]

Friend: *[Urgency in voice]*

> I call our Regional Biomedical Engineering Department.
>
> I leave a message on the answering machine
>
> Requesting one of the engineers return my call as soon as possible.
>
> I prefix my name with "Doctor" to ensure a response.
>
> I hate playing the "Doctor" card.
>
> But I've done it before.
>
> An engineer almost immediately returns my call.

[Speaks very rapidly]

> I quickly plead Ruth's story,
>
> Insisting that I'm not asking him to see Ruth ahead of someone else,
>
> Rather to see her after hours,
>
> And would be happy to pay him at an overtime rate,
>
> And would consider it a personal favour.

[Sheepishly]

> He jumps in before I embarrass myself further with,
>
> "Don't you think that every parent with financial means,

72

Whose child has cerebral palsy or a neuromuscular condition,

Offers to pay me to see their child after hours?

They all want their child in computerized education,

Rather than falling farther and farther behind kids their age.

Some parents without the money promise to 'beg, borrow, or

steal' to pay me.

I stopped returning phone calls two years ago.

The only reason I'm returning yours

Is because you're a physician."

Scene 18

[Lighting for bedroom at group home. Ruth flattens bed, removes hospital blanket and IV pole, and lies on her stomach facing audience.]

Ruth: Last week I developed another butt bedsore.

The nurse for the group home has me on my stomach all day

To expose my ass to the air.

Royal pain.

But I'll do anything to prevent it from getting infected.

Two years ago infection spread from a butt bedsore

Through my entire body.

By the time they got me to the ER

The doctors thought I was unconscious.

But I was just too weak from infection to open my eyes,

Or speak.

And of course I couldn't feel them pinching me,

So I couldn't respond to "painful stimuli."

But I could sure hear them all right.

Hear them debate my fate:

"Death with dignity" now,

Or a "persistent vegetative state" in their "expensive care unit,"

Possibly denying the ICU bed to someone

Who could recover with a higher "quality of life."

"Quality-of-life" assessment can trap people "like me"

In lethal traps.

[Ruth stands and walks to stage front.]

I really thought they were going to let me "die with dignity"

Right then and there;

Curtained off from help,

Where no one could hear my heart screaming

I want to live,

I want to live no matter what.

[Sits in memorial service chair Friend usually sits in]

Because the ER can be a very dangerous place for someone

"like me."

I considered having someone write me an "advance directive,"

Like I saw on Chicago Hope.

Except indicating the opposite:

I do want everything to be done to keep me alive,

No matter what.

Even "heroic measures."

But I heard there were problems with advance directives,

And began worrying that written words could be used

against me

To permit my "death with dignity."

Then I heard about "Life Story Decision Making."

You write down the names of people who know your life story

People who you trust to make decisions for you.

You need several names to ensure a few people can be

contacted

And corroborate each other's point of view.

Three women have already written their names and phone

numbers

On the special card in my wallet.

And I'm also going to ask my strange-doctor friend.

[Pause]

I know,

He doesn't know me very well.

And I don't think we've talked more than a dozen times.

But he was very upset when I told him about

The "death with dignity" debate in Emerg.

And he definitely knows I want to live no matter what.

And I believe his MD degree

Is my best defence against "death with dignity."

Doctors will listen to him when he tells them

She wants "to live no matter what."

He's a member of their club,

And doctors will have more trouble browbeating him

Than the women on my list,

One of whom has already written his name and phone numbers under hers.

I'll ask his permission next time I see him.

Scene 19

Friend: I wonder what it would cost to take Ruth to the States.

To get her hooked up to her computer there.

I know you can buy prompt healthcare in the States;

Why not biomedical engineer services?

I know if my children had to wait, I would find the money.

But Ruth is not my child.

She is my friend.

Anyway, I don't have time to take Ruth to the States.

No, that's a cop out.

I could hire one of the caregivers at Ruth's home to take her.

I'm sure they'd like to make some extra money on a day off.

They're only paid minimum wage.

Scene 20

[Group home lighting. Ruth sits in her chair.]

Ruth: The antibiotics resolved the bedsore after a few weeks,

And I've been great for months,

And I have something very important to tell you.

I am in love.

I am completely and so deeply in love.

I have found the soulmate I sought for so many years.

I know, soap opera clichés,

But I've hoped to feel them for so long.

[Walks to her desk]

I am so in love.

So Fuck'n A in Love

He listens to me so eagerly,

Longing to learn me.

He speaks to me so gently,

Calling me his calcedony,

Because he says I'm beautiful to the core,

Though a little crusty on the surface.

[Pause]

Okay, I showed him my bookends.

[Caresses bookends. Walks to stage front.]

I love the way he strokes the hair that sticks to my forehead,

Or moves my drinking straw to my lips when it goes amiss.

And the way he lovingly traces my jaw line to my chin.

With such soft, tender strokes.

Each caress of his fingers

Smoothes away years of loneliness.

I have never felt so alive.

His name is Alex but I call him Fred.

Fred had a stroke.

The left side of his body doesn't move.

He uses a chair,

But not a power chair like mine.

And even if he had a power chair,

He obviously wouldn't be able to go as fast as me.

But then few can.

Fred writes me poem after poem.

And he reads them so lovingly,

Although his speech is slurry.

I will write Fred poem after poem

As soon as I'm connected to my computer.

I will pour out the love collected in my heart,

The love bursting my heart

Every minute I am awake.

And I am so exquisitely awake.

Wait just one a sec,

An attendant's coming into my room.

[Whispers]

I'll tell you more about Fred later.

She says,

[Cheery voice]

"Ruth, good news.

An engineer's coming to see you on Tuesday

To assess you for your computer."

She smiles and leaves.

The word "assess" terrifies me.

What if my jaw muscles aren't working well enough anymore?

Scene 21

[Lighting for memorial service]

Friend: Another Friend lifts her eyes

And tells a story about helping "our Friend" smoke.

All smile, except me.

All eyes stare at me.

Encouraging me.

Waiting for me.

Waiting for me.

Scene 22

[Lighting for bedroom at group home. Ruth sits in her chair.]

Ruth: The biomedical engineer gently places my chin

Into a cold metal cup he calls a transducer.

It's connected by thin black and red wires to a little black box

That looks like a Geiger counter.

You know the things they use in old movies to test for radiation,

Little glass windshield over trembling red needle and all.

I don't hear any Geiger counter static though.

And I sure don't want to give this guy any static.

Heaven is in his hands.

I'm on my best behaviour.

I ask him if he thinks I'm hot.

Whoops.

He smiles and reminds me to only move my jaw when he asks.

He spends over an hour with me.

It's hard for me to be good that long.

As he gathers his stuff to leave I say,

[In a Rocky Balboa voice]

"Yo, Mr. Biomedical Engineer,

When do we hook up?"

He smiles, but apologetically.

"I'm sorry, you'll have to be patient."

Scene 23

[Ruth stands and walks to stage front and centre.]

Ruth: I've got another butt bedsore.

          The nurse has me lying on my stomach again all day.

          Ass-naked to the world.

          The worst part is I won't let Fred into my room.

          Not because I'm modest,

          But I'm sure the bedsore looks awful,

          And I'm worried it's starting to smell.

[Blackout]

Scene 24

[Ruth is lying flat on hospital bed with eyes shut. Friend stands holding briefcase and walks to desk. Night-time light or desk lamp on.]

Friend: I've just flown home from yet another conference.

Being away from my kids is hard,

And flying is claustrophobic.

But this time it was worth it.

A keynote speaker spoke softly into the microphone

The most powerful words I have ever heard.

She began by declaring,

Ruth: I am the healthiest person I know.

Friend: Which surprised the more than 500 attendees

Because she is quadriplegic.

She uses a state-of-the-art power wheelchair,

The seat of which periodically raises, lowers, and tilts,

To rotate pressure off the weight-bearing points on her skin.

She credits her wonderful health

To financial means and education,

Two of the World Health Organization's social determinants of

health

And most important,

Love:

The love of her partner in everything she does.

The love of her parents in insisting and financing the type of education

Where pages could be turned and doors opened,

Physically and metaphorically.

Her voice is now heard all over the world.

She writes by speaking into her computer,

Her words transcribed into text through software

I think she called "Dragon."

At the end of this amazing talk,

She read a list of names and causes of death

Of persons killed by government cutbacks to social programs:

A woman starved to death

Because funding for someone to check in on her was cut off

A man was burned to death

Because he was placed into a bathtub of scalding water

By a new and less costly attendant.

Many names and atrocities followed.

With each name, my heart heard a bell chime,

And saw a flame appear.

By the time she finished, the stage seemed carpeted

with candles

Of compassion,

[Chime]

Of equality,

[Chime]

Of purpose,

[Chime]

Of solidarity.

[Chime]

I have to tell Ruth about this amazing woman.

I haven't seen Ruth for a while.

[Walks across stage to desk looking tired]

No red light on my answering machine.

But there is a note from my 14-year-old son:

"The hospital called, going to bed."

I'm not on-call.

[Picks up phone]

I page the Clinical Fellow.

She's not looking for me.

Must be some confusion now rectified.

[Puts down receiver, takes off jacket, phone rings, picks up]

Hello.

Ruth: Ruth's in trouble,

Please come to the hospital right away.

[Dial tone]

Friend: *[Walks to stage front speaking rapidly]*

I quickly drive to the hospital,

Assuming the woman who called is on

Ruth's list of people,

Trusted to insist that all be done for her,

"No matter what."

I park illegally at the ER doors and dash in.

Ruth's not here.

At least she's been admitted.

I ask the receptionist where,

But her computer is taking too long.

I run up the stairs to Intensive Care.

The nurse at the desk is expecting me.

She looks frightened,

Says nothing,

But the index finger of her right hand

89

Is pointing to a draped-off area at the Unit's far end,

Where incandescent curtains project ominous shadows.

I turn to dash,

But she grips my right wrist,

Ruth: Why don't you stay here with me until they're finished?

Friend: I extricate my wrist and run.

I clench the curtain's edge and take a deep breath.

These drapes will not be Ruth's shrouds.

I fling open the curtains.

[Pause]

To horror.

Oh Ruth.

Bacteria have blackened her skin,

And swollen her body to a huge black balloon,

Knotted at her neck, elbows, and wrists

By a sadistic birthday party clown.

Ruth's closed eyes bulge like black tennis balls.

Her chin is gone.

I see a black Michelin Man.

The periphery of my underwater vision

Sees a woman sitting to the left of Ruth's bed,

Tears streaming down her face;

An ICU doc stands on my right,

Acknowledging me as he draws drugs into syringes.

Hollowness expands within me,

Vacuuming me downward.

I fight it.

I can stop this.

Ruth wants "to live no matter what."

I stare at Ruth,

Working hard to see,

Working hard to breathe,

Drowning in what I see.

I turn to the doctor.

You're not going to disconnect her?

He puts his hand on my shoulder.

He was once one of my students,

A Monday Night regular.

I tell him, Ruth wants to live no matter what.

He gently whispers, There's nothing left.

How can you be so sure?

He squeezes my right arm and says,

Look.

I put my body between Ruth's and his as

I'm supposed to do.

But instead of insisting that she remain on the ventilator,

I place my lips where Ruth's ear should be and plead,

Ruth, give me some sign.

Twitch an eyelid,

Something.

Please Ruth.

Please.

[Freezes under spot]

Scene 25

[Memorial service lights. Friend sits in same memorial service chair. He looks up and unfolds sheet of paper from his pocket.]

Friend: It's not Ruth's life that I can share,

For I knew little of Ruth's life.

And I can't share Ruth's death,

Too painful for me to recount.

But I can share Ruth's beauty,

That beamed in the sound bites I permitted her.

Ruth gave me so much,

Asked so little,

Received much less;

From me,

And from a health and social system

With limited capacity for compassion

And accommodation.

Her last words to me were,

I am in love,

Why don't you come on up and see me sometime,

And I'll tell you all about him.

Ruth was beautiful to her core,

Is beautiful to her core

Like the bookends that stood beside the computer

She was never permitted to use;

The bookends that now stand beside my computer.

[Light on Ruth who wears a peasant dress and sits in memorial service chair on other side.]

Ruth: He tells them her bookends are calcedonies:

Rough-surfaced rocks,

That can open to amethyst,

Agate,

Onyx,

Chrysoprase.

[Stands and walks to front of stage]

He tells them that each calcedony is unique.

That calcedonies have spiritual powers

Healing powers,

He tells them he will share her beauty.

He tells them he will always introduce her as my friend,

My friend who wanted to be a poet,

But is a poem.

My friend..

FINIS

Acknowledgements

I would like to thank Catherine Frazee for her inspiration, wisdom and encouragement. I would like to thank Lisa Balkan for her dramaturgical suggestions. I would also like to thank Sheila Boyd, Susan Cox, Les Friedman, Roxanne Mykitiuk, Jennifer Ryder, and Katharine Timmins.

Portions of Calcedonies were published in *Canadian Medical Association Journal*,[38] *From the Other Side of the Fence: Stories from Health Care Professionals* Pottersfield Press[39] and *Reflective Practice: International and Multidisciplinary Perspectives* Taylor & Francis,[40] and in whole in *Health and Humanities Reader* Rutgers University Press T. Jones, L. Friedman, D. Wear (Eds).[41]

---

[38] J.A. Nisker, Chalcedonies, *Canadian Medical Association Journal*, 2001, 164(1), 74-75.

[39] J. Nisker, Chalcedonies, In: Nisker J. (Ed.) From the Other Side of the Fence: Stories from Health Care Professionals. Halifax. *Pottersfield Press*, 2008, p. 172-176.

[40] J. Nisker, Calcedonies: Critical reflections on writing plays to engage citizens in health and social policy development. *Reflective Practice: International and Multidisciplinary Perspectives*, 2010, 11(4), 417–432.

[41] J. Nisker, Calcedonies. In: T. Jones, L. Friedman, D. Wear (Eds). Health and Humanities Reader. *Rutgers University Press*. (in press)

Sarah's Daughters

To the women we love who died of breast cancer
To the women who did not have to die from breast cancer
To their daughters

Characters

Joanne, a woman in her thirties or forties.
The performance also requires a cellist, a young woman, who plays between most scenes and gradually become a representation of future generations of daughters.

Act I, Scene 1

[Centre stage left is a rectangular table, representing a boardroom table. Surrounding the table are six chairs. On the table, in front of the stage left chair facing the audience lies a manila envelope and a black and white photograph. At the back of the stage stands a full-length mirror in a traditional dark frame. Back stage of the mirror is an open closet with costume changes that can be accessed throughout the production. In the closet will be a pullover dress, a blazer, some kerchiefs, some scarves, and several pairs of shoes. At stage right is a homey chair with a lamp table beside it. To the right of the lamp table sits a cellist. The cellist plays between each scene and as indicated in particular scenes.]

She lived with the knowledge it would happen to her,

Knowledge more felt than understood,

Knowledge gleaned from intuition that could not be confessed,

Knowledge that always lived but would never rest.

She lived with the knowledge it would happen to her,

Woke each day to the knowledge it would happen to her,

That what happened to her mother would happen to her.

She wondered only when it would happen,

When it would end.

[pauses]

When will it end?

When did it begin?

For me it begins with my grandmother,

Sarah,

With whom I lived at my life's beginning,

Who lived with us during her life's ending.

My wonderful second mother,

My first when my mother's care

Was younger brother shared.

[pauses]

My grandmother taught me so much:

Powdered in kitchen table flour,

She told stories of Schweitzer and

Hammarskjøld,

Patiently engraving her goodness,

To proxy me with the purpose

She knew she could not pursue.

[pauses]

Breast cancer found my grandmother when she was 45,

I was 15 when she died eight years later.

I did not know my grandmother had breast cancer,

I did not know she would die.

She suffered years of surgery, chemotherapy, fluid taps,

Carefully hidden behind parental backs

Forbidden to my focus.

[pauses]

But perhaps those backs were less opaque,

And it was I who chose to take

Each molecule of density to deny

Truth to a teenager,

Too enamoured with teenage rise

To be encumbered with adult decline.

[pauses]

Even when my grandmother lived in a hospital bed,

I denied where that bed led,

Till my mother's telephone whisper

"Joanne, Could you come to the hospital" insisted

It would be the last time.

Yet when my grandmother's eyes and mine entwined,

It was the first time they ever entwined in her truth.

[pauses]

I held her goodness in my hand

Long after "visitors' hours are now over"

Demanded I leave;

But I could not leave.

She would never leave while I held her hand.

It was my first joust with injustice,

I wore her colours,

I could not let her down.

I could not leave.

But "too young" rules decreed I must,

So I left, and lost,

And my trust of what was just

Was lanced forever.

[pauses]

I love my grandmother very much.

For years I grieved,

But never for one moment perceived,

That what happened to my grandmother

Would happen to her.

[walks to other side of stage]

It was six years later,

When that medical print premonisced

My mother would suffer the same injustice.

The fact soon fell from its suspended shelf,

My mother discovered her assassin herself,

Shortly after the mammogram I arranged

Proclaimed "all clear."

She bravely bore her long-accepted bier

And missioned to soften her family's fear.

[pauses]

Mastectomy delivered a tiny stone,

The surgeon delivered an optimistic poem:

There was no spread,

No further treatment to tread.

But the final pathology report

Delivered an "aggressive" retort

That was surgeon-shared only with the medical one.

[pauses]

It was a time,

It may still be a time,

When cancer patient families

Are encouraged to cheery possibilities;

Through tones that knell all's well.

So the doctor to nurse beware

Of all might not be well,

Was a care I did not share

With my now pastelled family.

I let her doctors take command.

[pauses]

The tumour's small size and negative nodes

Bode no tamoxifen, no radiation, no chemo.

Tamoxifen was new then,

It was thought that it might later lend

Leukemia

To women it borrowed from breast cancer.

Radiation and chemotherapy would hurl her further abuse,

I could not advocate their use,

Not when the surgeon's advice so soothed my family,

And me.

[pauses]

I abrogated my awareness,

Quiesced my mother to another's care,

And accepted a nursing job in California,

On a cancer ward.

Of course I now admonish this acceptance,

I should have shared her each remaining day

Finding ways to repay the love she lavished;

[pauses]

But there were no nursing jobs in Canada,

And a career turn would congeal concern,

Confess the poison she possessed,

So I left.

[pauses]

A year later,

My father's long distance words:

"I have some bad news,"

Collapsed my knees, my lungs, my life.

Nothing further was said,

She would soon be dead.

My silence heard my father urge

The already started chemotherapy would cure her,

A reassurance irrelevant to my mother's reality.

[walks to other side of stage]

As I flew home,

8 mm movies of my mother

Viewed each mile through invisible tears,

There were so many smiles in so few years.

No sound was needed to hear her embrace,

No colour required to feel her grace.

[pauses]

A friend once said my mother looked like Natalie Wood

In West Side Story.

I see my mother more beautiful:

On the dance floor,

Eyes smiling as she spins beneath my brother's arm

To meringue or swing,

Eyes in love as she folds into my father's arms

To "Love Is a Many Splendoured Thing."

I see her on the beach,

Eyes afraid as her children taunt Atlantic waves.

I see her at home,

Feeding my friends,

Who warm in the love of my mother's den.

[pauses]

I hurried the hospital's revolving door,

Then sped the elevator to the cancer floor,

Where doors open on black in-memoriam plaques

Engraving the names of the cancer-killed,

I did not pause to look for my grandmother's gold name

I could not help but see a black space below

Beckoning my mother's name.

[pauses]

I bolted to the nurses' station,

Breathlessly begging direction to her room;

I bolted into that room,

Only to find a woman who was not my mother

Smiling at me from a wheelchair.

I said "so sorry" and bolted next door

[pauses as if in door of room]

Before I was locked in abhor

That I had just spoken to my mother.

[pauses]

Panic punished as I tried to undo my betrayal.

I ran back to her room,

To her unvanquished smile,

To her "Don't worry that you didn't recognize me without

my hair."

I hugged her waist and begged her forgiveness.

She locked her fingers in my hair

And released me to her comfort.

[pauses]

With each week's advance,

My family firmed in their faith

That more chemotherapy could turn

Metastatic cancer's advance.

They were kindly encouraged to this credulity.

I knew no such luxury,

I silently shouldered death's answer,

While cancer poured its spores through my mother,

Growing tubes to drain its seditious sap

From her abdomen, her bladder, her brain, her back.

[pauses]

Soon the cancer that seeded her brain

Convulsed her body.

The doctors countered with sweet sedation

That dissolved her mind,

Taking her from us before we were ready.

I asked the drugs be backed off,

And that brought my mother back.

I'm not sure whether I asked that

For her or for us;

But her crystal comburence

Warmed one more cold month,

109

Till rare became the time she was aware

Of the love that surrounded her,

The love she put there.

[pauses]

My family still denied her imminent death,

And daily prescribed her doctors

Newspaper finds, such as Laetril

And other unevidenced medicinals of the time.

My gentle urge that no magic cures

Would miracle my mother,

Was met with silent haranguing

That my heart had been hardened in hospital training.

My mother began her terminal breathing pattern.

The elevator doors opened for the last time,

The "in loving memory" list embossed my loss.

My eyes tunnelled to resist seeing my grandmother's name,

My mother's name would soon join hers.

Then I felt my grandfather's arm eagerly effuse,

"Joanne, I heard about a drug on the news

That will soon be available to cure your mother."

I compassioned her death is immutable.

His helplessness tortured:

"Why do you think you know more than her doctors?"

I hugged him,

Then walked him to my uncle and aunt,

Pacing the verandah to the vigil

I would enter for the last time.

[pauses]

My father sat staring at his forever love,

Glad life would soon be over for her,

Sad love would soon be over for him.

My brother and I stood bookending her bed

Above the kerchiefed head we so loved.

Silent centurions,

Guarding the gates of the dead,

Prohibiting her pass.

I took my mother's left hand,

My brother took her right.

We were touching an angel's gossamer wings

As they slowly spread for flight.

As her final breath exhaled death,

My brother commenced cardiac massage.

I refrained his wrists in whispered gauze,

111

"It's okay,

She's gone but she will never leave us."

My eyes glazed.

I lifted them to my father's,

Searching mine.

We stared at each other for a long time,

Longing for her,

Allies in loss.

I held my mother's hand past cold.

I still it hold.

[pauses]

I love my grandmother very much.

I love my mother very much.

I look in the mirror;

And see a woman who is not my grandmother

Who is not my mother.

But who lives with the knowledge it will happen to her,

Knowledge more felt than understood,

Knowledge gleaned from intuition that could not be confessed,

Knowledge that always lives but will never rest.

She lives with the knowledge it will happen to her,

Wakes each day to the knowledge it will happen to her,

That what happened to her grandmother,

That what happened to her mother,

Will happen to her.

She wonders only when will it happen,

When will it end.

[pauses]

I have two daughters.

[pauses before cello music starts]

Act I, Scene 2

Linda.

I met Linda in the waiting circle

In front of our daughters' school.

Linda also has two daughters,

Linda also is a nurse.

[pauses]

Linda was the type of woman everyone noticed:

Everyone loved.

Happy. Excited, so beautiful.

Linda would smile to all the mothers

In our ritual pre-bell WAIT:

[sarcastically]

We wouldn't want to be late for our daughters.

But then she would linger at the car window

Of a pale thin woman

Who never left her car.

The woman always wore a kerchief

Around her sunken cheeks and tired eyes,

That would light up in love

When her son and daughter sprinted to her car.

114

[sadly and slowly]

Her children now slowly walk to the car of a man.

[pauses]

Linda now waits with me.

We never talk of the kerchiefed woman,

We talk about our daughters:

Their growth to almost womanhood

Our growth to definite parenthood.

[pauses]

We laughed at the coincidence

That two nurses would have a daughter named Sarah

The same age, at the same school.

My older daughter is Amy,

Linda's younger daughter is Jessica.

We didn't laugh at the coincidence

That our mothers both died from breast cancer,

Mine at 47,

Hers at 35.

I now know that the breast cancer

Is no more coincidence than the name Sarah,

Considering the school our daughters attend

Exists to extend them knowledge of the heritage

Their mothers' generation abandoned.

[walks to other side of stage]

Linda and I grew closer each week

Despite the commonalties of our past and present,

We are very different.

Linda has the quickest mind

[pauses]

And mouth.

[laughs]

I love listening to Linda think,

And you can truly hear Linda think;

Because her thoughts freely flow out her mouth,

Never filtered through a mask.

Linda leaves her mask in the garbage pail

Outside the operating room door.

Act I, Scene 3

[Sinister cello music plays. Joanne walks slowly over to table.]

An envelope and photograph float,

On a boardroom table,

Lifeboats on a glassy lake,

That remains smooth,

Though waves of fear of twenty years

Emanate from the envelope,

And from the white coats on the opposite shore.

[pauses]

The lake echoes no loon's soothing call,

No reflection of trees brilliant in fall,

Just the white coats,

And failing hopes,

For me,

For my daughters.

[pauses]

The lake remains smooth

Because two Halcyon women in the photograph,

Hugging eight-year-old me in the photograph,

Calm the waves with their warmth.

I focus on the photograph,

To keep my faith from lapsing

And allow the manila raft to come crashing toward me,

A death raft that can drown me.

[pauses]

I gently lift up my picture.

My fingers caress the bless

Of three women captured in love,

A grandmother,

Her daughter,

And her daughter.

Their love smiles love to the photographer,

My father, a wise man

Who so loves these three women:

His wife,

His wife's mother,

His daughter.

[pauses]

The table's gloss reflects the loss

Of my grandmother,

Of my mother,

118

Of my sisters;

Sisters not blood-related,

Not blood-related until perhaps

[pauses]

today.

Act I, Scene 4

When I was a nursing student,

A forty-year-old woman named Miriam

Handed me her genetic map to put in her hospital chart.

[Miriam's genetic family tree, as appears on title page, is projected or appears on blackboard or flip chart.]

Miriam called the shaded circles and open squares

Her family tree.

She said her doctor called it her pedigree.

[pauses]

Miriam's tree was truly sinister.

Dark circles hung like dead leaves.

Representing women dead from ovarian cancer,

That is all but one dark circle,

That woman died of breast cancer.

Every circle was shaded

Except Miriam's and her daughter's.

The square leaves were white

Meaning the men were well.

Miriam explained the trunk was short

Because previous generations died in the Holocaust.

Miriam was having her ovaries removed before they

became cancerous.

She asked if I thought she was overreacting.

Miriam was not overreacting.

[pauses]

Miriam was a lovely woman.

She showed me photographs of her son and daughter,

About my age then,

And a photograph of her dead mother

About my age now.

I reported to my instructor

Miriam's family history from Hell,

And her brave pursuit of prevention.

My instructor reported to me,

That the intern's routine "pre-op physical"

Declared Miriam would not have ovarian cancer on her

shaded circle.

[pauses]

It would read breast cancer.

Act I, Scene 5

Two years ago I heard on the news

That a Canadian scientist found the gene

That causes breast cancer in women my age,

And ovarian cancer.

I knew I was approaching the age

When our breasts become susceptible.

Linda didn't seem to know or care.

She said "There is always media hype over any cancer cure

The study is preliminary at best

Years of research will still be required

To be sure the gene's legit,

And to know how to use the gene's information

If it is legit."

[pauses]

"But Linda, what if B-R-C-A is the gene

That killed my mother

Or your mother,

Or both our mothers?"

[pauses]

"And if it is, Joanne,

What can we do about it?

No one can take it away."

[pauses]

Linda saw the BRCA gene's discovery

As a source of unnecessary worry.

I saw the BRCA gene's discovery

As a tool to prevent violation of my body.

You see I have contemplated preventative mastectomies

Every day since my mother's mastectomy.

Women with similar family histories

Were undergoing preventative mastectomies even then,

And I remembered Miriam.

I wasn't going to wait too long.

[pauses]

After I breastfed my youngest,

I booked an appointment to see a surgeon,

I was that ready.

But my marriage ended,

And as a single woman I saw mastectomies differently.

I worried no man could see my disfigurement,

Without seeing me as a disfigurement.

So I kept procrastinating the date.

Of course I would never admit any of this to Linda.

Act I, Scene 6

I am eight years old.

Foam falsies bounce from my mother's top dresser drawer,

With a little help;

As they have bounced many times before.

I love these falsies.

They are soft and squishy and capable of many games.

Like ricochet off the wall;

Like rhinoceros (one foam horn on forehead, another over

my nose);

Like the Tin Man in the Wizard of Oz with

One falsie serving nicely as his hat

And the other as his oil can.

I sometimes even use them as intended,

I am Wonder Woman.

I draw a lipstick star on my forehead.

Mostly I am my mother.

[pauses]

I once asked my mother why she wore the foam cones inside

her bra.

"Mommy, you have nice breasts already."

[pauses]

> She told me breastfeeding me and my brother shrunk her breasts,
>
> Just when someone named Marilyn made it the style to have large breasts.
>
> She said wearing the foam was just like wearing a hat.
>
> I want to look good for your father.

[pauses]

> I thought of my teenage breasts.
>
> The first time a boy touched them
>
> Through the armour of my not needed "training" bra,
>
> And my baggy, very much needed, thick sweater,
>
> So no one would know I didn't need a bra.
>
> The first time I allowed a boy to slip off my bra
>
> After eventually allowing me to unhook the clasps
>
> And not so gently caress my breasts,
>
> The first time a boy deliciously explored my nipples.
>
> And the first time a man I loved
>
> Caressed my breasts with his fingers and tongue,
>
> And love.

[pauses]

126

When I breastfed my daughters,

I felt the indelible meld

Of the nourishing love of my mother,

Jell-O chocolate pudding, Kraft Dinner,

Nestlé's Quik,

My mother's chicken soup

The love she ladled within her arms,

Upon her lap,

The love that still feeds me;

And of the sensual love of …

Not like when a man touches my breasts,

But still sensual.

I felt a oneness with the many generations of women

Who breastfed their babies love.

A oneness with many generations of women

Whose breasts were part of their sensuality.

[pauses]

I thought of my mother's breasts…

[darkens with cello]

[head turns to boardroom table]

Act I, Scene 7

[Joanne sits at table in same chair as before.]

The table is built for a board of eight

To counsel the fate of women like me,

Who soon will tune their lives to the envelope's core:

Who soon will be free,

Or absorb the sentence of generations of genes.

But today it seats just three,

My doctor, my genetic counsellor,

And me.

[pauses]

My kind doctor's compassionate voice,

Sprinkled with aware silences,

Shares the stairs I can climb

If I want to unwind

The code that might be sealed

Within the envelope,

Sealed within me.

I hear the doctor's professional words,

Professing cure

If the test censures my breasts.

Confident words,

Designed to dissolve fear in the goodness of knowledge.

He encourages I interrupt anytime,

Ask many questions,

But my answers are already there,

Within the envelope.

I find myself suddenly in no hurry for more knowledge.

I've waited 20 years for the knowledge

Now waiting for me

[pauses]

in the envelope.

[pauses]

I can wait a little longer to open its seal.

So I patiently wait for my kind doctor's script to end.

I patiently wait for my script to begin.

[pauses]

When he completes his speech,

I ask if he and my genetic counsellor would leave,

So that I might in privacy receive

What the test confessed;

So that I might in privacy grieve

The loss of my breasts, or death;

So that I might in privacy plead for my daughters.

Why must it happen to them?

Why again and again?

Act I, Scene 8

About a month after we heard the term BRCA,

I read a newspaper ad

Recruiting women who had a family history of breast cancer,

To participate in a research study of a test for BRCA.

[pauses]

I knew I had to volunteer immediately

And begged Linda to volunteer with me

"Just in case."

[pauses]

"I'll volunteer with you

Only because I have nothing to do tomorrow

After I drop off the girls

And you'll be too nervous to drive downtown yourself."

[pauses]

Linda drove us downtown to the hospital where my mother died.

I kept telling myself

We're only going here to volunteer.

We followed the signs to the research office,

Gave our names,

Filled out questionnaires,

And handed them back to the nurse.

[pauses]

> She looked at the questionnaires
>
> And proclaimed neither of us qualified for the test:
>
> No relative alive with breast cancer,
>
> And not enough relatives dead from breast cancer.
>
> She told us we could book mammograms.

[pauses]

> Just booking the mammogram's date
>
> Rakes my stomach in anticipation.
>
> As Linda and I drive downtown,
>
> I hope our not-so-young
>
> But still under-40 breasts
>
> Will tell the truth to mammogram film.
>
> My staccato speech betrayed my nervousness,
>
> Even though I know anything the mammogram reveals
>
> Will be concealed until our doctors' appointments
>
> Two weeks later.

[pauses]

> In the waiting room,
>
> My eyes survey the same Time magazine line
>
> With accelerating intensity.

I remember sitting beside my mother at her mammogram.

I wish my mother was here with me now

She would stroke my hair,

Tell me everything will be okay.

But at least Linda is here.

She respects my charade,

And keeps calling me Joanne

So I can't help know who I am.

[pauses]

The receptionist shouts "Joanne."

Why does the receptionist have to call so loud?

Everyone will know who I am.

I force myself to stand.

I feel like a clumsy elephant

As I try to move my body through the corridor.

[pauses]

I touch the narrow walls to the change room

Like a zombie in The Night of the Living Dead.

Am I the living dead?

[pauses]

My flesh is compressed

Under cold microscope glass,

My body leans forward and forward as commanded.

My breast is being ripped off.

It's no loss if it's ripped off.

I am being sucked into an escalator's cold teeth

As it descends into the floor.

There's a pause, then my other breast is bitten, and bitten.

I bite my tongue hard.

[pauses]

I hear "You're finished,

I hope it wasn't too unpleasant."

I slither back to the waiting room

To wait for Linda.

[pauses]

Soon Linda bounces into the waiting room,

Smiling,

Nonchalant,

[pauses, looks at audience]

Faking.

We drive home drained.

[pauses]

>I wait a week then call my doctor for the results.
>
>I know I wasn't supposed to.
>
>I know Linda wouldn't.
>
>But I had to know
>
>What my mammogram already knew.

[pauses]

>The secretary puts me through:
>
>"Nothing even suspicious."
>
>I thank his kindness and apologize for bothering him.

[pauses]

>I debate calling Linda to repeat the delicious words.
>
>"Nothing even suspicious."
>
>I know she would never call her doctor.
>
>She will know how neurotic I really am.
>
>But I want her to call her doctor,
>
>I want to be sure Linda's mammogram
>
>Saw "nothing even suspicious."
>
>I have to know Linda's safe.
>
>I can't wait.
>
>I call her.

Linda tells me I'm "nuts,"

And "no way" will she call

"If everyone calls their doctors for results,

Doctors will never have time to see patients."

I beg her,

She says, "Chill out."

But I sweat for two weeks.

Until Linda runs up to me in the waiting circle

And laughs "nothing suspicious"

We dance around like little girls.

Act I, Scene 9

One day Linda drives us to our mothers' cemetery,

To introduce each other to our mothers.

We talk to our mothers,

We laugh, we cry a bit.

Linda was only eight when her mother died.

She remembers her mother,

But not her mother's suffering.

Is that why Linda doesn't seem to fear breast cancer,

And I am terrified?

Act I, Scene 10

[Joanne puts on white coat and takes one of the boardroom chairs and moves it away from the table. She steps behind the boardroom chair and puts her hands on top, as if she is speaking behind a lectern. (A small lectern could be used instead.)]

The BRCA breast cancer gene

They call it BRCA

Is a specific sequence of 1,863 nucleic acids.

Insinuated in the 12th to 21st interval of the

17th chromosome.

It begins CGTAAC...

It has an autosomal dominant inheritance pattern

That means offspring have a 50% chance

Of having their parents' disease.

Now if a woman carries the BRCA gene

She has an 80% chance of developing breast cancer

In her 30s and 40s.

[pauses]

Scary?

Not really because this only applies

To women of Jewish ancestry

With a family history of breast cancer.

[pauses]

The vast majority of women

Who develop breast cancer

Are older women—most over 70 years of age.

And in these older women

It is likely that environmental factors

Rather than genetics

Are causative in this majority.

[Walks away from chair and takes white coat off.]

This Internet anecdote makes my enemy less mysterious

But not less dangerous.

I want to know my enemy.

[pauses]

If I carry a BRCA gene mutation

It insinuated itself into my life before my birth,

Where it quietly lurks until my thirties or forties

When it will transform my breast cells

To breast cancer cells.

It measures less than a millionth of a micron in diameter

But is the largest force in my life.

139

Act I, Scene 11

It is more than a year

Since Linda and I were denied the BRCA test.

It is cruel that I'm not permitted to its knowledge,

Knowledge that will either stop my worry,

Or quickly encourage me to have mastectomies.

[pauses]

But then logic intercedes and encourages

That even Jewish women

With family histories like mine,

Still have a 50-50 chance

Of NOT having BRCA gene mutations.

It seems extreme to seek mastectomies,

When I could wait for the BRCA test to be available.

Linda says, "If the test was that important

We would have access to it in Canada.

Like they do in the States

[pauses]

Okay, for five thousand dollars!"

I will wait with Linda.

Act I, Scene 12

We search the Internet for clues,

And conclude that breast self-examination

Is the best that we can do,

Except to hope.

So I hope and examine my breasts,

And hope with each palpation

That I will not find my death;

But Linda…

[speaks rapidly]

Her biopsy was immediately conclusive,

Mastectomy promised the elusive cure

Radiotherapy reassured.

Course after course of chemotherapy was endured

And tamoxifen was added just in case,

[pauses]

Because it's now safe.

[pauses]

Linda told me her tumour would eventually be tested for BRCA.

Act I, Scene 13

When Linda found her lump

I called my mother's oncologist

And begged he bestow my mother a wish,

That her daughter not suffer breast cancer,

But also not suffer unnecessary mastectomies.

I asked if he could kindly bend a branch of the BRCA study,

And send my blood for the test.

I begged him: "Pretend I have more relatives with breast cancer,

Because I would have more relatives with breast cancer

If the Holocaust had not killed my relatives."

I told him about Linda,

About how she could have been in the study

If Hitler's fires had not burned the leaves off her family tree

Our family tree.

[pauses]

The kind doctor immediately agreed

And gave me two aunts and one cousin

Dead from breast cancer

Yes, he lied for me.

Lied so I would live.

[pauses]

My blood was drawn to wait in racks

Of frozen reason for mastectomies.

The wait for its turn to be tested

[pauses]

Could be a year and a half!

I debate not waiting

I will have them off now!

[pauses]

Which fear is more powerful,

My fear of death

Or my fear of mutation?

Mutilation? Mutation?

I decide to hold off.

143

Act I, Scene 14

Another year goes by.

I wait for Linda's cancer to recur,

I wait for my blood to be tested for BRCA.

I dread losing them.

They're the most sensitive part of me.

I know they don't look beautiful anymore,

Two kids, each breastfed a year

(They say breastfeeding prevents breast cancer),

Anyway my breasts aren't firm or anything,

But they're still beautiful to me.

But if my test is positive

They become time bombs demanding disposal.

[pauses]

Linda is called in to receive her BRCA results.

She can't believe they tested her blood before mine.

She says "Joanne, you're the one who needs to know now,

It is too late for me to have preventative mastectomies."

[(cello music) walks to boardroom]

We wait outside a conference room,

[goes to boardroom table]

Whose open door reveals a boardroom table.

Soon Linda follows a doctor and a genetic counsellor inside.

I wait twenty minutes before Linda's tears

Declare BRCA positive.

I hug Linda.

We cry for her daughters.

Act I, Scene 15

I insist on accompanying Linda to all her medical visits,

I know she would insist on going with me.

I was there when the doctor confirmed

Linda's CAT scan's cancer recurrence in her liver,

On her ovaries,

Beneath her lungs.

[pauses]

Linda tolerated no consonant of camouflage,

No phrase of false hope.

[pauses]

When my mother had information to suffer

We would buffer the information

Through a well practised eye language.

My mother always understood.

Act I, Scene 16

[sits at table]

I do not see the white coats leave,

Just hear the click of my closed door.

I do not care what will happen to me.

It is what will happen to my daughters

That takes me to the room's far corner,

That takes me to my knees

To pray to the women who pray for me.

Like a Shintoist I pray to their picture,

I whisper an ancestral prayer

That I have whispered so many times before;

But today I must be careful

Not to crease their caress with my tremble,

Not to smear their smiles with my tears.

I ask for their love,

Their sustaining love.

[pauses]

I wait.

Then feel their hands on my shoulders,

Feel them firming my shoulders,

Firming my spirit not to hide,

Firming my body to rise,

To return their faces to the glossy surface,

[pauses]

To pick up the envelope's purpose,

Which I still pretend is to set me free,

Though I know that can never be.

Act I, Scene 17

[stands and moves one step from table]

Linda opts for more surgery,

Then more surgery.

Then more chemotherapy.

Then more chemotherapy.

[pauses]

Linda says "When breast cancer took my hair it took my identity."

Cancer tries to take away her identity,

But Linda is still Linda.

[pauses]

She fights to become well enough

To pick up her daughters from school.

She succeeds.

She comes each day wearing a brightly coloured kerchief

With polka dots, or rainbows, or smiley faces.

I stand by her car every day,

Talking to Linda

Through the car window.

[pauses]

Act I, Scene 18

I stare at the envelope

[pauses]

I had asked my kind doctor

To loan me a sample test report,

So I could learn where the punch line lurked,

So when today came,

My eyes would find the punch line first

And quench knowing's thirst as soon as possible,

For what was possible for my life,

For what was possible for the lives of my daughters.

[pauses]

I pick up the envelope,

I inhale a deep breath,

I exhale "Get it over with."

"Accept it."

I open the envelope.

I draw the report from its scabbard.

I close my eyes.

I unfold the verdict.

I open my eyes.

The punch line pummels what I always knew it would say:

[pauses]

Positive for BRCA.

[pauses]

Not that there's any disbelief,

There's even relief that the gene test proves

What I already knew:

Death by breast cancer if I do not remove my breasts.

But at least the declaration is complete,

I will soon sleep,

And not wake each day wondering

Will it happen to me?

Then I think of my daughters and collapse,

My mothers try to hold me up.

But they can't

They allow my new tears to blend with old.

I fold the paper back into its manila tomb.

[pauses]

Will what happened to my grandmother,

What happened to my mother

What will happen to me

Happen to them?

I stuff our curse

Down to the bottom of my purse.

I feel like a bad mother,

An abusive mother,

For bringing them here.

Act II, Scene 1

It took ten months before I could get an appointment with a
surgeon.

It may take another ten before my name

Claims top spot on his OR list.

I am trapped behind a dissolving bulletproof vest,

Is it not cruel to make me wait?

To have my fate fulfilled

When I could erase my fate tomorrow?

Act II, Scene 2

Linda found a lump on her head,

And then another.

One remained pea size,

The other quickly developed into a robin's egg.

She feels them when she thinks we're not watching.

We try not to watch her feel them.

My mother developed lumps on her head.

One was a plastic reservoir

Whose tubes shunted fluid off her brain.

The many others were cancer like Linda's.

[pauses]

Again I call my kind doctor.

Again I beg he intercede,

And plead my case to the surgeon.

He says there's nothing he can do.

[pauses]

I need them off. Now!

While there's still time.

I don't want my children to watch me die.

Like Linda's children are watching her die.

Like I watched my mother die.

Act II, Scene 3

[Joanne covers the boardroom table in a royal blue tablecloth and places the candelabra in the centre. She sits at the table in the same chair as in boardroom scenes in Act I.]

While I wait, we celebrate Sarah's bat mitzvah,

And celebration plans distract me.

I even forget to palpate them some days.

[pauses]

I'm so glad the celebration is now.

I still have them,

And Linda is still alive

To share her magic tonight.

[pauses]

As my Sarah turns from child to woman,

My knowledge of BRCA burns,

Like the candle on Sarah's cake

She lights to commemorate her great-grandmother,

Like the candle Sarah lights to commemorate her grandmother;

Like the candle Sarah lights in love for me.

If my surgery would only happen soon

Sarah will never see me struggle

Like Linda struggles at the next table.

[pauses]

When Linda walked into the banquet hall,

A hand on each daughter's shoulder,

Her husband cautiously close behind,

She smiled at me,

Linda's perfect sparkling smile,

That still surfaces

From the sunken cheeks and sallow skin

That a make-up artist tried to glow with health

An hour ago.

[pauses]

People who don't know Linda,

Still know what she must have,

Even though she wears a wig tonight.

I hear people whisper:

"Who's that?"

"That can't be Linda!"

I "shush,"

I don't want her to hear

That even in her carefully chosen wig,

She no longer looks like Linda.

For tonight is for Linda.

Sarah will be cast in other parties,

This is Linda's last.

[pauses]

I look at the throng of 13-year-old wrigglers,

Most are Sarah's school friends,

Their heritage is our heritage.

I try to halt my horror

As I wonder who of these happily dancing girls

Dance with BRCA alterations

Hidden under their dresses?

Who of these girls will one day have mastectomies?

[pauses]

Should I warn their mothers?

[pauses]

Now Linda, strong as always in her will

Is on the dance floor,

Holding her daughters' hands

While the DJ blasts Britney Spears.

The next song starts "Oh my love, my darling…"

And Linda's husband asks if she's taken for this dance

Linda smiles yes and hugs him.

157

They gently sway together

Like one willow in a soft breeze.

There are no tears,

The dance is sacred,

The dance is goodbye.

[pauses]

I refocus on my daughter's night;

And turn beneath my brother's arm

To Ricky Martin and Swing Kings.

I am filled with joy for my daughter,

I abandon Linda,

I abandon me,

I abandon our legacy.

Act II, Scene 4

How do I tell my daughters?

I consulted a child psychologist, who said,

"Wait as long as possible before broaching the subject.

Why encumber more of your daughters' years

With fear of losing breasts that are just developing,

Why alter their sense of womanhood?

[pauses]

But there's more to womanhood than breasts.

And is their youth an excuse

To defer the truth of our cancer,

Till they quilt their own answer

From scraps of conversation or press,

Or pendulums of my happiness.

Will my body's disfigure carve runnels for their fear,

Unnecessary fear for one or even both of them?

[pauses]

I'm afraid my daughters will find out themselves.

Recently there was a TV show on BRCA,

That I surreptitiously prevented them from watching.

But more TV will come,

And my daughters will criticize

My lack of confidence in them.

They've developed that teen tendency

Of insisting on the truth.

Act II, Scene 5

July 19, 2001

I lie on Linda's bed as we watch the 11 o'clock news. All days are bad now. The anchor announces that tomorrow's *New* England Journal of Medicine will report a three-year follow-up on BRCA testing in the Netherlands. 160 women in the study tested positive for BRCA gene mutations. None of the 93 women who had preventative mastectomies developed breast cancer. Of the 67 women who declined mastectomy, seven have already developed breast cancer.

[pauses]

August 11, 2001

Myriad Biotech Corp of Salt Lake City claims it holds the patent on the BRCA gene test and demands Canadian provinces pay $3800 for each woman tested in Canadian hospitals, or face legal action.

[pauses]

August 25, 2001

The province of British Columbia stops BRCA gene testing.

[pauses]

August 26, 2001

Linda dies.

Act II, Scene 6

A stream of slow moving cars

Lake behind a black iron gate.

Foreign letters wrought over the gate

Forge German sounding words,

Though the letters are Hebrew.

I have always cringed at this gate,

Because words canopied over another gate,

Arbeit macht frei,

Mark the entrance to another place

Where Jewish women remain forever.

[pauses]

Though Linda's bones will not be heaped for bulldozer burial,

Linda's flesh was not starved by anti-Semitic hate,

But she did starve to death;

And though her emaciated face never stood behind barbed wire,

Her face is as familiar.

[pauses]

Linda's daughters follow their mother's casket,

Carried by eight men selected by Linda,

Her brother, three cousins, four friends,

162

Men who may be selected by BRCA,

To unknowingly carry breast cancer to their daughters.

I cry because of their daughters,

And Linda's daughters, and my daughters.

[pauses]

The tableau for our dead is posed.

Ancient words are said:

Yis gadol va yis kadesh

I whispered the words at my grandmother's funeral,

Yis gadol va yis kadesh

I whispered these words at my mother's funeral.

Yis gadol va yis kadesh

I whisper these words today

Because I owe my life also to Linda.

Her coffin slowly sinks to the earth.

[watches as coffin lowers]

I take my daughters' hands

And join the heavy-footed trickle to our cars.

[pauses]

As we approach the gate

An invisible colander prohibits our pass.

The pores that allow other mourners to flow through

Are somehow too small for us.

I ask my daughters,

"Do you want to visit your grandmother?

And my grandmother?"

They both have wanted to come here with me many times before,

But I have always come alone.

I never wanted them to see me cry.

I never wanted them to consider that I might die

And lie here beside my mothers;

Their tears withhold words,

Their eyes say yes.

[pauses]

My daughters and I turn toward where we've been.

We pass where Linda lies

Next to her mother

[pauses]

But my eyes are fixed a hundred yards away,

On two pink granite headstones,

Beckoning us side by side.

[pauses]

As we approach their headstones,

We see flowers spreading beneath

Like two shimmering aprons of spring:

My father still sends flowers to the women he loves.

I start to softly cry.

My daughters cry when they see me cry.

I cry harder.

[pauses]

I kneel before the polished pink headstones.

I caress the poem of their smooth permanence

With ritual strokes of my hands.

Then I lovingly lift the silver oval covers

That protect the faces of my protectors.

"This is the last photograph of your great-grandmother,"

"This is the last photograph of your grandmother."

My daughters are pained by the sadness in these photographs.

Much healthier pictures of these women

Pillar our dining room door.

"Your great-grandmother's picture

Was taken at your uncle's Bar Mitzvah,

She was very sick,

She thought she wouldn't live to that day.

Your grandmother's picture was taken at my wedding.

[pauses]

We had to move up the date so she would live to that day.

They're wearing wigs."

My daughters sob harder.

[pauses]

My index fingers ritually trace

The loving letters carved in the stone

That spell my mother's name,

That spell my grandmother's name.

Names carved on memorial plaques in the hospital,

Where three months ago

They helped me pass to safety.

[walks to other side of stage]

I had told my daughters I had cysts in my breasts,

And my latest mammogram suggested

They might become cancer one day,

So my doctor suggested rather than live afraid,

I should take off my breasts.

I told my daughters it was easy to agree

Because my breasts don't define me as a woman,

Why should they confine me in fear?

166

[pauses]

I didn't tell them the truth

I didn't tell them the about BRCA,

About what it means for them.

[pauses]

I had not been to the cemetery since my mastectomies.

I found excuses like recuperating,

Like giving more time to Linda.

Why do I feel guilty for avoiding breast cancer?

[pauses]

Then I look at my daughters

And I feel the guilt I truly should feel,

The guilt of passing on this BRCA gene

To one of my daughters,

And they don't know this.

[kneels, shivering and retching, gasping for breath]

My daughters are frightened.

They try to calm me

I plead for my mothers' help.

Because I can't live with the knowledge it could happen to them

Wake each day to the knowledge it could happen to them!

Please Mommy, tell me when to tell them!

Please Bubie tell me how to tell them!

[pauses]

My daughters don't know how long to let me cry,

I don't know how long they let me cry,

Before I feel my daughters' hands on my shoulders,

Feel them firming my shoulders,

Firming me to rise,

To return to them.

I hug them hard.

[pauses]

It is always difficult for me to close the cover on my mothers' faces.

I always kiss them goodbye first,

Cry, kiss them goodbye again.

But I can't close the covers today.

I stare at my mother's picture,

I stare at my grandmother's picture.

I stare at my mother's eyes,

I stare at my grandmother's eyes;

[pauses]

I realize they are speaking to me,

[pauses]

> They are telling me it's okay to tell my daughters,
>
> My mothers are telling me
>
> They will help me tell my daughters
>
> Yes, we will tell them together.

[pauses]

> Though the ground is still damp,
>
> I ask my daughters to sit with me,
>
> Where I have sat so many times alone
>
> To receive my two mothers' goodness.
>
> I look up at their pictures
>
> I feel their eyes encourage me.
>
> I inhale their wisdom.
>
> I inhale their love.

[pauses]

> "This is your great-grandmother,
>
> She is wonderful.
>
> This is your grandmother,
>
> She is wonderful.
>
> They both died from breast cancer,
>
> But I will not.
>
> Nor will you.

From Calcedonies to Orchids

[pauses]

Do you know what a gene is?"

FINIS

Acknowledgements

I would to thank Liza Balkan and Kayla Gordon for their dramaturgical assistance, as well as Genome Canada and the Ontario Genomics Institute for funding the original production tour.

Portions of *Sarah's Daughters* were published in *Ars Medica* University of Toronto Press.[42]

Optional score by Alyssa Wright is available from jeff.nisker@lhsc.on.ca

---

[42] J. Nisker, She lived with the knowledge, *Ars Medica*, 2004, 1(1), 75–80.

A Child on Her Mind

with Vangie Bergum

In memory of Kit Benson, RN

Characters

Jane, a woman in her thirties.

Moira, a nurse in her forties or fifties.

Eva, a woman in her twenties, who physically resembles Carol Cameron.

Carol Cameron, a 40-year-old woman.

Stacey, a 16-year-old woman.

Jeannine, a 16-year-old woman.

Act I, Scene 1

[The set consists of three birthing rooms. Eva and Carol occupy one, Stacey and Jeannine another, and Jane is alone in the third. The lights come up on Eva and Carol's room. Beside Eva sits Carol, expensively attired in a pale blue silk blouse and complementary tights. Spot on Jane.]

Jane: I have always wanted a baby. It's part of life. I'm not saying a woman who doesn't have a child is missing something from her life. But I've always known if I didn't have a child, I would be missing something from mine. It took me a while—I wanted a career, independence—but when I got to be thirty, and I know this sounds clichéd, it was almost a biological clock thing. I hadn't done anything about having a child. But when I finally became pregnant, even though I had sore breasts and felt morning sickness, I still carried the possibility that I wasn't really pregnant, that there really wasn't anything in me, that I had made up pregnancy symptoms because I wanted to be pregnant so badly. When I felt my baby move, move within me, it was the first time that I allowed myself to believe that I actually was going to have a child after all. Feeling my baby move made me recognize it as a child, and made me recognize what having a child truly means. At that moment, my life changed forever. I felt vulnerable.

[Nurse Moira enters, gowned in greens and white Converse running shoes. She reads from and writes on a clipboard.]

Moira: Hello, Jane. My name is Moira. I'm your nurse for his shift.

[They shake hands.]

Jane: I'm very pleased to meet you, Moira.

Moira: Jane, when did your contractions start?

Jane: Oh, about six hours ago. I'm not really sure, they just kind of crept up on me.

Moira: Let's hope they keep creeping.

[Spot on Eva.]

Eva: *[speaks with a thick Slavic accent]*

My life was wonderful before war come to our village. The door to our home open on poem of pine trees, atticing sunlight on our stream. I dream, I dream the dreams of a girl on the stream's warm bank. When I older I thank God for being woman on that bank, when Valon, my lover—my husband—when Valon and I drink our bodies' beauty by that stream. And after we make love we look up to moonlit mountains, whose serated summits starred our sky, starred our lives. Until the soldiers scarred our skies with smoke from their guns, scarred our lives with their war, took Valon's life from mine forever.

[Moira enters Eva's room.]

Moira: Hello—

[looks at chart at foot of bed for name]

       Eva.

[picks up chart]

       My name is Moira. I am your nurse for this shift.

[She offers Eva her hand but as Eva stares straight ahead, Carol takes Moira's hand across the bed and shakes it professionally.]

Carol: My name is Carol Cameron. I'm her labour coach. I am here

       to help in any way I can.

Moira: Eva, when did your contractions start?

Carol: Moira, she doesn't speak English. She's asked me to answer

       for her.

Moira: We can get an interpreter.

Carol: No, she understands English. She just doesn't speak English.

       So an interpreter won't be necessary.

Moira: Okay. But it is my responsibility to inform you that the

       hospital will provide an interpreter at any time if you don't

       understand my questions

[pauses]

       or Carol's answers.

Carol: She's absolutely sure.

[Spot on Eva.]

Eva: My name is Yvanka Magdorjevitch, but when I come to

Canada, Mrs. Cameron call me Eva. I call her Mrs.

Cameron, always Mrs. Cameron, until one year ago, when

Mrs. Cameron ask me to call her Carol, when Mrs. Cameron

ask me to call her friend.

Moira: And don't be afraid, Eva, we are all your friends here.

Eva: But I can never be Mrs. Cameron's friend. Even when I no

longer working for Mrs. Cameron, she will always be my

employer. That can never end.

*[Stacey sits up in her bed, with Jeannine sitting in a chair beside her.
Moira enters Stacey's room.]*

Moira: Hello—

[looks at chart at foot of bed]

Stacey. My name is Moira. I'm your nurse for this shift.

[shakes Stacey's hand]

Stacey: Moira. Cool name, Nursey. Can you believe this is really

happening? Too cool!

Moira: Of course it is, Stacey.

[still looks at clipboard but indicates Jeannine]

And who is this?

Stacey: Jeannine, of course.

Jeannine: Hi. I'm Stacey's labour coach.

Stacey: Jeannine's going through this with me, through the whole

thing with me, right Jeannine?

Jeannine: I'm with you to the end, Stacey.

[Spot on Jeannine.]

Stacey chose me to be her labour coach because I'm her best
friend. She counts on me, not her boyfriend, not her mom.
She doesn't get along with her mom. She doesn't get along
with her boyfriend for that matter. But Stacey's great. Pure
energy and joy.

Act I, Scene 2

[Stacey, Eva, and Jane all have a contraction. Moira enters Jane's room.]

Moira: That was a great contraction, Jane.

Jane: That's wonderful. I'd really like to have a natural birth if possible. Intervention frightens me.

Moira: How quickly are your contractions coming?

Jane: I think they're about five minutes apart now. You'll have to ask my husband. He's in charge of timing contractions. He just went down to the cafeteria for a coffee but he'll be right back. He doesn't want to miss a thing.

Moira: Jane, it says your last menstrual period started September 17?

Jane: That's about right.

Moira: Are your menses regular?

Jane: Well, when I'm on the pill they are.

Moira: And you stopped taking birth control pills when you wanted to get pregnant?

Jane: Yes...

[Spot on Jane.]

Jane: I must admit I'm afraid of the pain. So far it's not been so bad. I think I can get through it. I've read so much about the pain of childbirth, pain disguised in euphemisms like contractions or rushes. Funny, I'm really worried about being noisy. I don't want to be yelling, out of control. But if you believe birth is a natural process, then it will happen more naturally.

[Moira enters Eva's room.]

Moira: How fast are the contractions coming, Eva?

Carol: About every five and a half minutes now, much stronger and more regular over the last half hour.

[Eva grimaces slightly as she controls a contraction.]

Moira: That's a great contraction, Eva.

Carol: I think she's developing an optimal labour pattern, don't you, Moira?

Eva: Two years ago Mrs. Cameron sponsor me to come to Canada. I thank her for that. Things very bad in Kosovo. There is war there. There is hate there. There is such cruelty there. I owe her much.

Moira: Let's wait for this "optimal" contraction to pass before I go.

Eva: But how do I know how much I owe? How much I owe to not still be in Kosovo with the soldiers? How far must I go before debt is forgot?

Moira: Eva, it says here that your last menstrual period started September 14.

Carol: That's correct, Moira.

Moira: And were your menstrual periods regular, Eva?

Carol: Yes, quite regular and we're quite certain the calculated date of confinement is correct. She is at term now, Moira.

Moira: And how are you so certain?

Carol: She told me when conception occurred. Does the doctor know we're here?

Eva: I happy like all children in our village. But I more lucky. My mother teach me to read. I love to read, and read all day on riverbank. Of course, this before I love Valon on riverbank. When Valon and I lie on riverbank, I have child on my mind even then. We dream of carrying child in backpack up those mountains that smile on our village. We dream of our child's smile when we look down on our home, the home we would one day build near stream.

[Moira enters Stacey's room.]

Moira: There are a few questions from the admission history I'd like
         to clarify, Stacey.

Stacey: Clarify away. . . Cool-Name-Nursey.

Moira: When was your last menstrual period?

Stacey: I think—it was in September, right Jeannine?

Moira: Could you be more precise?

Stacey: Like what?

Moira: Like, when in September?

Stacey: I don't know. Ask Jeannine.

Moira: And how would Jeannine know?

Stacey: Jeannine knows everything. She's the smartest kid in the whole
         school.

Jeannine: It started September 13th.

Moira: Are your periods regular, Stacey?

Stacey: Oh yeah, like a clock, not like Jeannine here. She never knows
         when her period will come. Mine comes like a fuckin' alarm
         clock.

Jeannine: My Mom doesn't like me spending so much time with Stacey. She tries not to say it, but she thinks it all the time; Stacey is a bad influence that hanging with Stacey will deprive me of being a doctor or a scientist or a writer—something that matters. But Stacey needs me. There is no one else there for her. Her mom's always busy with boyfriends, and she doesn't see her dad more than twice a year. I mean, my parents aren't perfect either, but at least they're always there for me.

Act I, Scene 3

[Moira enters Jane's room.]

Moira: So, Jane, do you have any medical problems?

Jane: No, I'm completely healthy now.

Moira: Jane, have you smoked cigarettes or used alcohol during the pregnancy?

Jane: I never smoked, Moira. My husband and I used to share a bottle of wine at the end of the day, but I stopped completely when I got pregnant. Are there any TV sets between here and the coffee shop?

Moira: Yes, several.

Jane: Is there a Leafs game on tonight?

Moira: I'm not sure.

Jane: My husband wants this baby as much as I do. He really is supportive of me. I want my husband to go through this experience with me, but I understand how hard it is for him to see me in pain. I also understand how hard it is for him to miss a Leafs game.

[Moira enters Eva's room.]

Eva: I glad when I see agency ad to work in Canada. I say choose
           me, please choose me. And I lucky, agency choose me. I
           mean, Mrs. Cameron choose me.

Moira: Have you had any medical problems, Eva?

Carol: No medical problems. She has always been in very good health.

Moira: And how do you know that?

Carol: From—I know everything about her. She is my friend.

Eva: Then I answer "yes" to Mrs. Cameron's contract, to be her
           housekeeper in Canada, to be safe from soldier attack.

Moira: Are you sure you don't want an interpreter, Eva?

Eva: I come to Canada. I comply with Mrs. Cameron's wishes, I
           clean her house, I wash her dishes, I iron her clothes. I
           content to cocoon two years of my life as Mrs. Cameron's
           domestic, a sanctioned servitude I would undertake to
           metamorphose into Canadian citizen, a free woman, never
           again to fear.

Moira: Eva, have you been on any medications during the pregnancy?

Carol: She was on no medications other than vitamins, of course. We
           started folic acid three months before conception and added
           iron and other vitamins at approximately twenty weeks
           gestation.

Eva: A year ago, when Mrs. Cameron ask me to call her Carol, to call her friend, my servitude was sentenced to never end. I see that evening forever. Mrs. Cameron call me to her living room. The room sparkle with silver and crystal vases; but there no flowers in vases. Mrs. Cameron ask me to drink wine with her. She never before ask I drink wine. Now she ask I drink wine from crystal glass, glass I always wash carefully by hand, after she warn me never put in dishwasher.

Moira: Have you smoked or drunk alcohol during the pregnancy?

Carol: Of course not, Nurse.

Moira: Eva, it says that you have had no other pregnancies?

Carol: That's right, Moira. When is our doctor coming?

Eva: The night Mrs. Cameron ask me to call her friend, to drink her wine, I saw the crystal and silver for the first time, as ornaments to add worth to her life when she show friends. Now she want me to add worth to her life, to give her something else of value to show friends.

[Moira enters Stacey's room.]

Moira: Stacey, have you had any medical problems?

Stacey: No I never got sick till I got pregnant. Not like Jeannine here. She's so sugary sweet every bug that goes by lands on her. Right, Jeannine?

Moira: But you became sick during pregnancy?

Stacey: Of course, doesn't everybody, you know that morning sickness shit.

Moira: Stacey—

Stacey: I puked my guts out every day for three months. I couldn't go to school. Jeannine came over to cheer me up, but my boyfriend never cared. He thinks puking is cool.

Moira: Stacey, have you been on any medications during the pregnancy?

Stacey: Well, there was this vitamin shit the doctor said to take right away,

[laughs]

some acid thing, right, Jeannine?

Jeannine: Folic acid.

Stacey: Yeah. And then there were these other vitamins I started back in September. They really bung you up.

Moira: It's the iron. Keeps your hemoglobin up, dear.

Stacey: Whatever. They make you shit bricks.

Moira: Really, Stacey.

Stacey: *[laughs]*

        Bricks of iron.

Moira: Stacey …

Stacey: It's true. I think they put it in the pills so you can practise pushing the baby out.

Jeannine: When I got back from Montreal the whole school was talking about this girl Stacey being pregnant. I didn't really know Stacey, even though we'd always gone to the same school. Then one day I walked into the bathroom and saw her frozen, just staring at the mirror. I didn't know what to do. I touched her arm and she started to cry. She told me her mother's boyfriend wanted her to have an abortion, and when she told him where to go, he called her a filthy little slut. Then she turned to me and said, "That's when I decided I'm keeping my baby." I thought she was the bravest girl in school.

Moira: Stacey, have you been smoking during your pregnancy, or—

Stacey: Gee, Nurse, back off! You think I would do anything to harm my baby? Just because I was stupid and got pregnant doesn't mean I'm stupid. And you know, I've been smoking since I was twelve. It was really hard to give up my butts. Just ask Jeannine. But I did it.

Moira: And Stacey, have you had previous pregnancies?

Stacey: Yeah, when I was eight! Give me a break, Nursey! I'm only 16.

Jeannine: When Stacey found out she was pregnant she was cool about it, but people are mean to teens who get pregnant. When Stacey told her mother she was pregnant, her mother's boyfriend demanded she have an abortion. That is, her mother's last boyfriend. Who did he think he was? What gives people the right to tell you what to do with your baby?

Act I, Scene 4

Jane: I always wanted to have a baby, the years of trying, of crying, hurled hollowness through the soul of someone who always considered herself lucky, lucky to be alive. When I missed my period completely, I was so excited. I thought I was pregnant.

Moira: It says here Jane, that you gained twenty-eight pounds during your pregnancy.

Jane: Yes. I've been eating a very good diet, and keeping myself fit.

Eva: Everything pretend change. Mrs. Cameron always cold, but now she warm and kind. Then Mrs. Cameron tell me about child on her mind.

Moira: It says you gained thirty-two pounds during this pregnancy, Eva?

Carol: Yes. I made sure she ate very well.

Jeannine: There's no easy way out of being pregnant. You have to think about abortion, about adoption, you have to think about keeping. There's no easy way out.

Moira: It says here that you gained thirty pounds during your pregnancy?

Stacey: Yeah. I've been a blimp for months. You know, it's amazing—where does all that extra skin come from?

Jeff Nisker

[Lights change to focus on Eva, Jane, and Jeannine.]

Eva: When Mrs. Cameron ask me to carry her child, at first I not know what she mean. I think she maybe adopting a child. I care for her child or maybe carry that child in my arms. I not sure. My English as you know not good. I not know that she want me to be mother of her child.

Jeannine: When I told my boyfriend I was pregnant, all he said was it must be a mistake. He was the mistake. He said he would wear a condom. He said a lot of things, like I was the most beautiful girl he had ever seen, like he loved me. Like he would never leave me. I chased after him for a bit but couldn't stand myself, so I just said, "Forget it. I don't need this."

Jane: The pregnancy test was negative. And my period never came again. Over the next few months I repeated the pregnancy test over and over. And it always read, no baby. I went to my doctor. He was really surprised my period had stopped. After all I was only thirty-two.

193

Eva: Mrs. Cameron try to embrace me with her eyes, but I know there no kindness in her heart. So I keep my eyes low. When I no longer can look down, I look away from Mrs. Cameron's eyes and see myself framed in her carved silver mirror, the mirror that hangs over her carved marble mantel. I see simple woman mired in middle of complex web.

Jeannine: I agreed with my mom to have an abortion. We cried. She said, "Let's just forget about this, we'll get out of this situation and things will go back to normal. We'll be just as happy as we were before."

Jane: When I told my doctor I wanted to become pregnant, he referred me to a fertility clinic. It took four months to get an appointment. I waited. I worried.

Eva: I afraid. I shiver under her pretend-warm eyes. Then Mrs. Cameron put her arm around my shoulder. My body go rigid. I feel her flesh through her blue silk blouse, burn through my red cotton dress, brand my flesh, make me her slave. Mrs. Cameron then ask again I do favour as friend, I give her child that God not send.

Jeannine: I couldn't do it. My mother cares about me a lot, but she cares about herself, too, and about how her friends would see that her perfect family wasn't so perfect after all. I had embarrassed her. Let her down. But I couldn't do what she wanted.

Jane: When I finally walked through the fertility clinic's doors I was greeted by hundreds of baby pictures smiling along the happy corridors. There was a huge photo collage of babies conceived within the clinic's walls. The further I walked along the clinic's corridors, the more my confidence increased. And when I took off my coat, I was so optimistic, I actually smiled. I said, come on, doctor, find out where my periods went and give me the drugs to bring them back, because I am really going to have a child. I must have a child.

Eva: Mrs. Cameron explain that Clinic lawyer would give contract. After I sign contract Mrs. Cameron said I could stop working for her as maid but continue to be paid. Carol think I have no problem comply with her wishes. To Carol I am creature whose hands do her dishes, whose womb would soon contain her child.

Jeannine: So my mother called my aunt in Montreal. Explained her "embarrassing" situation—my embarrassing situation—and asked if my aunt could help us out. She wanted me to go to Montreal so no one would ever know that I was pregnant. That I was a bad girl. That I was dumb.

Jane: The doctor shook our hands and told us not to worry, the clinic helps hundreds of couples like us have babies every year. He sent my husband off to produce a sperm sample. As the doctor continued his questions, his optimism grew delicious and I gratefully drank it in.

Eva: Mrs. Cameron's contract would be written in the highest moral ink, I would not have to have sex with her husband. His sperm they collect in doctor's office, cleanse under doctor's care, and transfer to my womb through doctor's sterile instrument. She not say that if I not sign contract she send me back to Kosovo, say I not good housekeeper, not fulfil my first contract. But I hear her threat. I know Mrs. Cameron. She get what she wants.

Jane: Then the doctor asked about past illnesses. I told him about the leukemia I had when I was nine, how it was cured by chemotherapy. Concern immediately betrayed his smile. He no longer seemed confident. A nurse took me to an examining room and asked me to get undressed. I waited. The doctor examined me, his voice reassuring me as he took his swabs. Then he handed me a requisition for blood tests and told me to come back in six weeks. Jeannine: My mother told me to tell my friends that I was going to Montreal to become completely bilingual. I guess she wanted to protect me, but I really didn't think it would be a problem at school. Well, maybe the teachers wouldn't think I was the perfect student anymore, but the kids would be okay with it. I mean, look at Stacey. She's doing okay.

Eva: I hear myself say "yes" to Carol's request. Her thank you took my soul from me. I hang my head when I hang my coat in Clinic corridor, close my mind when I close change room door, strip off my dignity as I strip off my clothes, and freeze my heart as I put my heels into cold steel that spread my legs to allow more cold steel to penetrate my soul. And as Carol's husband's sperm was injected in my womb, my soul was infected forever.

Jane: For six weeks the doctor's concerned look burned away my optimism. I should be grateful for chemotherapy. It saved my life. But now the doctor was telling me that the chemotherapy that saved me had also destroyed half of my ovaries' eggs. And now the rest had run out. I would have had children right after we got married if I knew my eggs would run out. I just thought get the house paid off, advance my career a bit, get a few holidays out of my system, then have a child. But the child was always most important. Nobody told me. Nobody told me I'd run out of eggs. I guess nobody knew then.

Act I, Scene 5

Carol: I'm an insurance executive. I design corporate plans for some of our country's largest companies. I'm forty. You might think that's a little old to be having a child, but I've just never had time. I always knew I'd have a child, a daughter to be precise, that I would call Katherine. I went through life doing what I was supposed to do, taking the talents I was given, adding lots of determination and working my way up the corporate ladder. My child had to wait. And as I began to soar in the corporate world, I knew that if I stalled my career climb to have a baby the stall would be permanent. I've seen other careers crash with motherhood. You see, if I took time out for pregnancy, when I returned I would have to work under the men who now work for me. I'm close to the top of the ladder but not close enough. I just couldn't let a pregnancy consume my business plan. Well, by the time I was thirty-eight, a child was definitely on my mind, so I decided, biological clock tick and all, I had better initiate my child plan. I thought it would be easy. But my clock was running faster than I thought. After a year of temperature charting and ritual right-day-of-the-month sex, I went to the Fertility Clinic. Their tests said I was running out of eggs.

My "age." Not being able to have a child was the first time in my life I couldn't achieve what I wanted through hard work and brains. It wasn't fair. There were options. Adoption? Could take forever. International adoption. I wanted the baby to look like me. Fertility drugs? In vitro fertilization? I don't have the time. But their next option, surrogate pregnancy, interested me. I wouldn't have to take the time to deal with IVF drugs or surgery, or even get pregnant. The downtime from work would be minimal. It sounded perfect. The clinic lawyer said the best bet for a surrogate would be to sponsor a woman from Eastern Europe to work as my housekeeper and later ask her to be impregnated with my husband's sperm instead of housekeeping. Apparently there were Eastern European women who, after being sponsored to Canada as domestics, would rather bear my child than wash my windows. The Clinic lawyer had arranged several of these "gestational arrangements" already this year. I studied the surrogate catalogue. That is, the catalogue of women applying to come to Canada as domestics. I found Eva. She was well-read for that part of the world, therefore probably bright. But I must admit my main attraction to her was her physical attraction, okay, her resemblance to me, not only in her face but in body. I was sure she had all the genetic traits that would translate into my child.

Eva: I was defiled by steel three times. I was infected by sperm three times, before I miss my period, before pregnancy test confess I carry this child.

Jane: I would not be a failure. I told the doctor to give me whatever fertility drugs I needed, to use whatever technology he had, anything. I wanted a baby.

Jeannine: I went to Montreal so I wouldn't have to have an abortion. I didn't want to hurt my parents, so I agreed to give the baby up for adoption and get on with my life. It was the hardest decision I ever had to make.

Eva: I have no voice, I had no choice but to sign the consent to lend Carol my body, bend to her wish to make me her chattel, her chattel for a child.

Jane: Now I carry this child, this wonderful child.

Eva: Now I carry this child, this wonderful child.
Jeannine: Now…

Act I, Scene 6

[Lights change. Moira with a due date wheel.]

Moira: Did you have an ultrasound?

Carol: Yes, at twelve weeks.

Stacey: Yeah, was it ever cool!

Jane: Yes, at twelve weeks.

Moira: When, Stacey?

Stacey: When, Jeannine?

Jeannine: At twelve weeks.

Moira: What did the ultrasound say?

Jane: That my baby was doing well.

Carol: The child was 12 weeks. You know, length consistent with dates, heart rate regular, everything normal.

Stacey: I dunno. They spread this gooey gunk all over.

Moira: Stacey—

Stacey: It was cold as Hell and tickled too. I laughed so much I almost peed.

Moira: Stacey—

Stacey: Well, my bladder was full.

Jeannine: I didn't really believe it was happening. Even when I saw my baby on the screen, it was still hard for me to accept that I was really pregnant. But the ultrasound made my baby more there.

Jane: The ultrasound really brought the baby into focus for me. Even though you'd think the baby was a separate being, somehow, the ultrasound just confirmed my feelings that we were one entity.

Moira: Are you sure you don't want an interpreter, Eva?

Carol: Thank you for your concern. She'll be fine.

Moira: Do you remember when you first felt the baby move?

Jane: Yes, January 19. It was a Saturday, I was just about to fall asleep, and then I felt it. I knew for sure what it was. I was ecstatic!

Moira: Do you remember when you first felt the baby move, Stacey?

Stacey: Do I ever! It was like...wow...Jeannine, wasn't it about the same time I started those vitamins back in January? It was a Saturday. Remember, Jeannine, we were watching TV at my place, that is, my mom's place, and all of a sudden I feel this bump. At first I didn't know what it was. I thought it was gas. But somehow Jeannine knew, knew it was my baby moving.

Act I, Scene 7

[Moira enters Eva's room.]

Moira: That's another contraction coming, Eva. You're doing very well. Do you remember when you first felt the baby move?

Carol: Yes, it was January 29th, 4:15 p.m. It was just a subtle flutter under my hand.

Moira: *[turning the due date wheel]*

No, it is when Eva first felt the baby move that helps us confirm dates.

Carol: We know the exact dates of conception so we don't need these questions. But she felt the baby move the same day as me.

Eva: I feel baby move two weeks before Carol. I not tell her. I want to have time when child would be all mine, when I could feel child swim within me, speak to my heart without hearing Carol's voice. My baby and I shared this wonderful secret, this secret wonder.

Jane: When I felt the baby move it became real, it suddenly became real. Until then, I couldn't allow myself to believe this was happening. We had tried so hard for so very long, but feeling the baby move made it all real.

Jeannine: When I felt my baby move inside of me I became less and
less sure I could give her up. My baby became more and
more real to me. I kept telling myself it belonged to someone
else, that I was helping someone else out.

[Contractions begin. Moira enters Stacey's room.]

*[Stacey gasps, begins panting in rehearsed Lamaze patterns. It is soon
obvious she has skipped most of the classes. Jeannine has pulled up the
sleeve of her sweatshirt to expose a large watch and is counting silently
to herself while her eyes flit from Stacey back to the watch.]*

Moira: Stacey, how quickly are your contractions coming?

Stacey: *[in pain]*

I don't know. It's hard to tell when you're in Hell. Ask
Jeannine.

Jeannine: It's been five minutes.

[Moira enters Eva's room.]

Eva: I cringe when Carol touch my abdomen. It is like she suck my
child's goodness out with her hand, take possession of my
child before it is even born, take my child to be her child
before I am ready.

Moira: How quickly are your contractions coming, Eva?

Carol: Every two minutes and thirty seconds. Shouldn't we have a fetal monitor hooked up so that we can watch the baby's heart rate continuously?

Moira: Carol, we're listening to the heart rate with a doptone and there doesn't seem to be a problem. If we put a fetal monitor on, Eva will have to stay in bed and she might want to walk around during labour.

Carol: But isn't a fetal monitor the most accurate way of knowing if the baby's healthy? It monitors the heart rate at all times. What if the baby's in trouble? We won't know until the next time someone comes around to listen to the heart rate. I really think we should have the monitor.

Moira: The doctor was here just an hour ago. He doesn't think it's necessary.

Carol: You want the monitor, don't you, Eva?

Eva: Carol insert verbs into every sentence of my life, verbs to ensure the baby be perfect. She supervise my meals, my vitamins, my exercise. She make sure I go to sleep early. But I only pretend to sleep. I lie awake to feel my baby move, breathe, beat, while I still can.

[Moira enters Stacey's room.]

Moira: Are they becoming very painful, Stacey?

Stacey: Painful! The last one was fucking hell.

Moira: Let's keep calm.

Stacey: Calm!

[pauses; smiles]

> That's why Jeannine's here. She'll keep me calm if anyone
>
> can. Right, Jeannine? Shit! Another one's coming!

Jeannine: OK, OK—I'm here for you, Stacey. You're doing great.

[Moira enters Jane's room. A contraction comes. Jane has a more difficult time with this one, but is still in control. Moira unobtrusively checks her watch.]

Jane: *[coming off contraction]*

> I guess it's going to get tougher before it gets easier?

Moira: Well, that was quite a hard contraction. You're doing very
          well but there's a long way to go. Would you like an
          epidural?

Jane: No!—I'm sorry, I'm not convinced they're safe.

Moira: They are quite safe, I assure you.

Jane: I don't trust drugs.

[gasps]

> I really want a natural birth.

[Moira enters Stacey's room.]

Stacey: *[still gasping as the contraction comes to an end]*

Hey Nurse! This pain really sucks! Aren't I supposed to get drugs or something?

Moira: Well, I could ask for an epidural, Stacey, or even some analgesics for the pain, if you wish.

Stacey: Yes! Both!

[gasps]

What are you waiting for—Elvis? Get the shit quick!

[pauses]

Act I, Scene 8

Moira: I chose nursing to help people. I chose obstetrical nursing
because of the beauty of childbirth, the beauty of helping
women become mothers. I really was a good nurse once.
Hard to believe. I would hang around long after my shift was
over if one of the women in my care was about to deliver, if
one of my babies was about to be born. The nurse coming on
would have to urge me out saying "It's my turn!" My
patients sent me thank you cards often framing a picture of
babies named "Moira." Babies named Moira. What a thing.
Now I'm just running from room to room, never really
connecting with the woman in the room. They're all a blur,
an amalgam that I struggle through each shift. It's almost
comical how I ricochet from room to room, never sitting
down, never inviting confidence, never being a shoulder to
share pain, to unburden fear. I feel like the silver ball tilting
in a pinball machine. Top score at the end of the day
determined by the number of patients I convey from labour
to delivery;

[pauses]

rather than a good day determined by how I helped women become mothers. How I helped this amazing process.

[pauses]

My focus is on information and machines. It's been a while since someone sent me a picture of a "new baby Moira."

Act I, Scene 9

[Moira enters Eva's room.]

Moira: This is quite a hard contraction, Eva. You're doing very well, but your cervix is just ripening now and there is a long way to go. Would you like an epidural to take away the pain?

Carol: Wait a second. I've read that epidurals increase the chance of forceps delivery. I do not want the child to be damaged by forceps.

Moira: But there's such a long way to go, and I know Eva's in a lot of pain, no matter how she tries to conceal it.

Carol: She has a high pain tolerance.

Moira: I'm glad you think so, but even still …

Carol: No epidural, right Eva? We only want what's best for the baby.

Moira: Well, what about a narcotic injection?

Carol: Don't they stop the baby from breathing?

Moira: It will wear off long before birth.

Carol: What if there's fetal distress and a Caesarean section is needed immediately! The baby won't be able to breathe when it's born!

Moira: We'll handle it. Eva, there's still a long way to go. Are you sure you don't want an epidural or at least some analgesics?

Carol: No! Remember, she speaks very poor English.

Moira: Eva—

Carol: No! I assure you she has a high pain tolerance.

Eva: Carol's house has beautiful nursery. Over the beautiful white crib, brightly coloured animals dangle on tiny threads from music wheel. When Carol not home I sit in rocking chair beside crib and gently rock to music as animals ride around their carousel. I feel baby move in me. I feel baby move me. I stare at crib and know one day my baby will lie there and Carol watch from rocking chair and Carol hear music. But never will feel music as I do, will never feel love as I do.

Moira: Are you sure you wouldn't like an interpreter, Eva?

Carol: No.

[Stacey and Jane speak simultaneously.]

Stacey: Shit, here comes another contraction!

Jeannine: Stacey ...

Stacey: Oh shit! Shit!

Jeannine: Stacey ...

Stacey: Jeannine, do something!

Jeannine: I can't.

Stacey: Where's that fuckin' nurse!

Jeannine: Stacey, I can't

[Jeannine runs out.]

Stacey: Jeannine ...!

[Jane takes Lamaze breaths.]

Moira: I'm not sure you understand, Eva. We can take away your suffering.

Carol: No, she understands. Isn't that right? You do understand.

Eva: I do understand. I understand more than Carol understand. I understand that as my child grow within me, the fact that I agree to concede my child to another makes me unfit mother, will always make me unfit mother. I feel I degrade my child. I feel I sell my child. Even though I have no choice to be mother of my child. I have no choice not to be mother of my child.

Carol: You do understand?

Eva: I understand more than I understand when I sign Carol's contract. But then just as now, I have no voice.

[Blackout.]

INTERMISSION

Act II, Scene 1

[Spot on Moira.]

Moira: I had a case last night. Silently shouting for my help. I wanted Eva to look at me, to talk to me, to shout "help me!" I could palpate her need. But why did I insist that she plead in words, what she was already pleading with her soul? I have two children. They're 12 and 10. I love them so much. Having gone through childbirth myself allows me to know my patients' needs. After all, patients today are the same as when I had my children. But nurses are different today. I'm as good a mother as I can be. I'm as good a nurse as I can be. But I used to be a much better nurse, much like the nurses who cared for me, who were aware of how I felt, how painful the contractions really were, of how I was becoming exhausted pushing my baby out. They encouraged, they compassioned, they shared personal stories of women giving birth. I used to do that. Now I have to pull in my antennae so I won't feel what I don't have time to feel. And when sense subtle, or not so subtle situations, that require extra care, that require compassion, I have to raise my time-efficiency shield, well-trained to protect me from subtleties. Keeping things safe is all I have time for.

214

Act II, Scene 2

[A three-bed postpartum room. One bed is empty, where Stacey would be. Jane sits smiling, reading a book on breastfeeding, and Eva sits in her bed, staring stonily straight ahead. Jane notices Eva's distress and her eyes move from the book to Eva and back, and again to Eva, who still stares ahead, not noticing Jane. Jane tries to make eye contact with Eva. Finally Jane sets down her book, gets up, and walks across the room.]

Jane: Hi. My name is Jane. I must have been asleep when they

         wheeled you in. Having a baby is hard work. Tires you out.

[pauses]

         Is everything okay?

[pauses]

         Could I help you in some way?

[pauses. Eva continues staring away from Jane.]

         I'm sorry. I guess everything didn't go well with your birth.

[Eva continues staring.]

         Is your baby okay?

[Eva looks straight ahead as she speaks.]

Eva: Baby okay.

[pauses]

         I think she okay. I no see her today.

Jane: You had a daughter. I had—have a daughter too. Aren't our babies wonderful? When mine came out, she opened her eyes and had a very long look at me, very intelligently— almost as if she recognized my voice. . . What's your daughter's name?

Eva: I don't know.

Jane: You'll come up with a name soon.

Eva: No.

Jane: Well, I have a name book somewhere you can borrow, if that would be helpful. I see your name's Eva. That's a nice ame.

Eva: My name's Yvanka.

Jane: I'm sorry, it says Eva on your bed.

Eva: Carol call me Eva.

Jane: Carol?

[Eva stares.]

I've heard that often women feel down after they give birth. I mean, the excitement pushes our adrenaline level up and when it goes down, well, some of us feel down for a while— the postpartum blues, they call it.

[pauses]

We'll all be smiling soon when we take our babies home.

216

Eva: I no take my baby home.

Jane: I'm sorry, I'm so insensitive. You're giving your baby up for adoption?

[Eva stares.]

I know it's none of my business. But you should feel good about yourself. By giving your baby up for adoption, you're giving a wonderful gift to another woman.

Eva: I not give. Carol take.

Jane: Carol?

[Eva stares.]

Eva, you can change your mind up to 30 days after the baby is born.

Eva: Too late. I already sign. I no can change mind.

Jane: But if you don't want to give your baby away no law can make you.

Eva: You no understand—

Act II, Scene 3

[Stacey bounces into the room, bounces on her bed, excitement flowing from her eyes, and bounces over to the foot of Eva's bed.]

Stacey: Wow! I just came from the nursery. The babies are just too cute. Eva, yours is the star. You can tell her from the nursery window. She has so much black hair.

Jane: Stacey, I don't think Eva is feeling very well. It's sometimes difficult the first day after having a baby.

Stacey: Eva, she looks just like you.

Jane: Stacey, could you do us a favour and go to the nurses' station and get another box of breast pads? I think our cupboard is bare.

Stacey: Okay, Jane, I'll be right back. See ya soon, Eva.

[Stacey exits.]

Jane: Eva, you're giving a precious gift to another woman. She'll be good to your daughter, she'll give her a good home.

Eva: You no understand.

Jane: I do understand. For the longest time I couldn't have a child. I tried everything: fertility drugs, IVF procedures, everything failed. My ovaries are basically dead. When nothing worked, my husband and I decided to adopt.

Act II, Scene 4

[Jeannine appears in spotlight.]

Jeannine: When I first went to Montreal it wasn't so bad. My aunt was

sympathetic and supportive. She took me to a teen

pregnancy clinic. The nurses and doctor there were as

respectful of a fifteen-year-old as anyone could be. They

talked to me about my options. Giving the baby up or

keeping it.

Jane: My husband and I decided to adopt. The lawyer told us we

were good candidates for adoptive parents. We had good

incomes. We bought a nice house near a school, three

bedrooms, big backyard, and waited for the adoption

agency's home study. And waited. And waited.

Jeannine: I kept thinking of my options — to give it up or to keep it. But

I didn't really have any options. I owed it to my baby to

give her the best home possible.

Jane: There were many times we wanted to get out of that waiting

cage, sell our family-to-come lifestyle and be free-spirited,

you know, condo, travelling, exotic sports, social functions.

But we didn't. We stayed surrounded by the white picket

fence, in the family house near the school, near children. Poised to have children.

Jeannine: I had a picture in my head, you know: white picket fence. Since I couldn't provide the white fence or the home within its warmth, I had to find parents who could.

Jane: Finally our home study came. I was evaluated for two whole hours. I was on trial, at their mercy: I was so careful to say what would make me a perfect mother. I was terrified they would disqualify me from motherhood.

Jeannine: The Clinic set me up with a private adoption agency that would ensure my baby be adopted by good parents, parents who could provide good things for my child. Parents I could choose from a catalogue.

Jane: I prepared my file so carefully. I must have drafted the "Dear Birth Mother" letter a hundred times, then revised it, and revised it again, trying over and over, line by line, to anticipate what the birth mother would want to hear, to assure her that I would be the best mother for her child.

Jeannine: I tiptoed through the files, but none of the couples caught me. No white picket fences. I was frustrated. I couldn't find the perfect mother. I wouldn't be a perfect mother either. But I could try.

Jane: I tried hard to be young enough, old enough, financially secure enough, down-to-earth enough, conservative enough, liberal enough, committed enough, religious enough, appreciative enough. I tried to show her that I was what she wanted me to be. Every day I waited for the agency's call. I laid my whole life on the line in that file. I opened my heart. And I was rejected.

Jeannine: I kept looking for the mother I wanted for my baby. The mother I wanted to be.

Jane: They said my file had been shown twenty times. Which means that I was rejected as a mother twenty times.

Jeannine: Then I opened her file and looked at her picture. Such a nice smile. I read the "Dear Birth Mother" letter. She said she knew what a hard choice I was making, and that she would do whatever she could do to help me stay part of my child's life. She seemed so honest and kind, and understanding of me. She said that she had always wanted a child, that it was the most important part of her life, that she would always do what was best for my baby.

Jane: Then one day the agency called. We were selected. The social worker warned that the birth mother might change her mind and decide to keep the baby. She said that happens a quarter of the time. But I was still ecstatic.

Jeannine: The agency suggested we meet in a restaurant. You know, anonymous, non-threatening, that sort of thing. I phoned the couple and asked to meet them.

Jane: The birthmother called and asked that we meet in a restaurant.

Jeannine: My mother went with me. I was nervous. Really nervous. They seemed nervous too.

Jane: I was nervous. And grateful. And nervous. I had tears running down my cheeks. I couldn't stop thanking her.

Jeannine: The adopting mother was so happy to see me, so grateful to me for choosing her.

Jane: I wanted so much just to touch the baby under her heart, the child I hoped would be mine.

Jeannine: She thanked me over and over for choosing her and promised to be the best mother she could be.

Jane: But I was afraid to come too close. I tried not to say my baby. It was always the baby. I kept telling myself I could lose my child.

Jeannine: She said that I could see the baby any time I wanted to, that she would help me out. I guess she meant financially.

Jane: There were a lot of things I wondered about but couldn't ask. Like did she smoke, or drink, or take drugs? The answers wouldn't have changed anything.

Jeannine: I had questions written down. They had questions written down. And we just asked each other questions. It went really well.

Jane: She seemed level-headed, steady, an average teenager in a situation she wasn't ready for.

Jeannine: After the meeting, I phoned them, they phoned me. We kept checking each other out. I couldn't help wondering about this couple. Were they the best I could find for my baby? I wanted the best—the very best.

Jane: When the baby was born, my husband and I went to the hospital with flowers. We went every day with flowers, and saw her, and saw the baby. She would let me hold the baby — my baby.

Jeannine: Before the baby was born I tried not to think of it as my baby, that kind of thing, so it would be easier to give up. I kept thinking I'm doing this for someone else. I'm helping someone else. But then when my baby was born, I really felt it was my child. It scared me.

Jane: I could see it was hard for her. Every day it seemed to be getting harder and harder for her.

Jeannine: I didn't want to hold her, to feel closer to her than I already felt. I knew it would make giving her up even harder.

Jane: I was getting really panicky because I thought the longer they were in the hospital together, the closer they were getting.

Jeannine: When the social worker asked me to sign the papers, she told me I had a month to change my mind.

Jane: She signed the papers at 9:30 the morning she was to be discharged. We were at the hospital at noon, but at four o'clock she still hadn't gone. I wasn't sure what was wrong. Was she ill? Was she having second thoughts?

Jeannine: The adoptive parents knew I was having second thoughts. They came and saw me that day, and told me they knew. I asked them how could they tell? And they said just by looking at me. But even though I was having second thoughts, I knew my child would still be going home with them.

Jane: Finally they told us we could take the baby home. When my husband brought the car seat up, we both lost it.

Jeannine: I could see them through the window of the nursery. I watched them leaving with her. I watched them go into the elevator. I went into the nursery. My baby's crib was still warm.

Jane: It was so cold outside. We bundled her up. She was so precious.

Jeannine: I went back to my room and looked out the window. I saw her waiting for the car. The last thing I saw was her fixing the blanket on my baby, making sure she was comfortable.

Jane: When we got her home I thought, okay, now it's all just a technicality. We just have to wait the month.

Jeannine: Everyone wanted me to give my baby up, so I did. But it was so hard. I just kept telling myself, "Do the right thing. Do the right thing. Don't be selfish. Do the right thing."

Jane: That month, I felt like I was at everyone's mercy, not just the birthmother's, everyone's. And then the lawyer called and said that the teenager had changed her mind. The lawyer felt maybe if she came to our house and saw the child was being well looked after, she might rethink her decision. So they asked her to pick the child up at our house. She brought a friend with her. And when she saw the child, she cried and kept saying that she was so sorry, she was so sorry.

Jeannine: I did what I was supposed to do. I did the right thing.

Jane: It was as if my child had died.

Jeannine: My child is almost nine months old. I haven't seen her since she left the hospital. I wonder what she looks like, what she's doing. What she's feeling. I know she's being cared for, being loved. But she calls someone else "mummy." Yet I'm her mummy, too. I'll always be her mummy.

Jane: I couldn't go through adoption again.

Act II, Scene 5

[Lights back to postpartum room.]

Eva: But Jane, why adoption? You have this wonderful baby of your own ...

Jane: Yes ... Another woman helped me. Gave me her eggs, so I could have a baby, too.

Eva: Gave you ...?

Jane: They call it egg donation. The Fertility Clinic found a woman to donate her eggs, someone who was infertile like me but didn't have the money to pay for her own IVF treatment. We paid the $6,000 for her IVF, and she gave me half her eggs. The Clinic fertilized the eggs with my husband's sperm, and placed the embryos in my uterus. One of them made it, and now I have my very own baby.

Eva: Did she have baby too?

Jane: I don't know. Maybe. I don't know who she is, it's all done anonymously.

Eva: So this woman maybe not have baby ...?

Jane: I don't know.

Eva: You take her baby ...?

Jane: No, it's my —

Eva: You take her baby, just like Carol take my baby.

Jane: Eva, you can have another child.

Eva: That what Carol say. But Carol take my daughter before the pregnancy test positive, before I see her on ultrasound machine, before I feel her move in me. I had no choice but to sign contract because Carol would send me back. Things very bad in Kosovo. I no want go back, but now I wish I never sign contract. I love my baby. I want to keep my baby. I wish I never sign contract. I wish I never leave Kosovo. I must give baby to Carol. I sign contract.

Jane: You mean, like a surrogate contract?

Eva: Yes, surrogate contract, I sign. My child now not mine. I lose my child to Carol like woman lose her child to you.

Jane: I don't think — I'm sorry Eva. I'm sorry for your loss.

[Jane exits.]

Act II, Scene 6

[Jeannine enters.]

Jeannine: Is this Stacey's — are you okay?

Eva: I wanted to hold her so much. But I couldn't. The nurse look
          at me as if I bad mother because I shake my head when she
          give me daughter to hold. But although I try not to look at
          her when I bring her to our world, I feel my love grow a
          thousandfold and feel my pain grow a thousandfold.

[Moira enters holding a baby.]

Moira: Eva, if you've made a mistake, you can take your child back.
          You have a month to change your mind. Your baby …

Eva: Once I put my arms around her, I can never let her go. I leave
          hospital today. I will never hold her.

Moira: Eva, let me help you.

Eva: You no understand.

[looks at baby]

          If I take my child back, I must go back

[pauses; dawning as to what she must do]

          to Kosova.

Moira: You're right, Eva. I don't understand. If you think you can be

a better mother to your child than Carol, why give her up?

[Eva turns to Moira. Their eyes meet. Stacey re-enters, brimming with breast pads and baby.]

Stacey: Jeannine! You came back!

Jeannine: Stacey, I'm so sorry —

[Stacey hugs her.]

Stacey: Hey, no sweat.

[shows Jeannine her baby]

Well?

Jeannine: Stacey, your baby looks just like you.

Stacey: Well she will once she gets some piercing done.

[pauses]

Just kidding!

Jeannine: Stacey, there's something —

Stacey: I can't wait to take my daughter home to my new apartment. It

might be small, but it's all mine, mine and my baby's. And

that's just too cool.

[Fade out of postpartum room to soliloquy lights.]

Act II, Scene 7

Jeannine: I couldn't do what Stacey's doing—let a baby deprive me of my life. But I know why she's keeping her baby. It's probably the first time in Stacey's life that someone will really love her unconditionally. Although it will be hard for Stacey, I think Stacey will feel better about herself than she ever has. She will pour every molecule of herself into her baby. I know I couldn't do it.

Stacey: At first it was really cool. Everyone tellin' me how cute my baby was, how much my baby looks like me. But after a few crying nights it wasn't much fun anymore. And my boyfriend's no help. Macho man. He thinks he's so great because his dick made this kid. But while he's out bragging to the boys, I'm stuck at home changing diapers, complaining to the TV. Last week we went to the beach. My boyfriend lit out for the pier with the boys, while was stuck in the hot truck breastfeeding. When I'm finished I ask him if he'd just take the baby for a few minutes, you know, give me a chance to go in the water and cool off. And he says sure, and holds her up for the guys to see. But by the time I get my bathing suit on, he's had enough. He gives the baby back to me and says that he has something important to do, then disappears in one of his buddies' cars, probably to a bar somewhere. All I hoped was they card his ass. My mother — Thank heavens for Jeannine. She's the best mother.

Jane: I heard a TV journalist call egg sharing "bartering" for eggs. She said that it might become illegal as it commodifies human tissue. That it's coercion of an infertile woman into giving up half her eggs, which reduces her chance of having a child. But is it coercion? She would have had no chance of a child without my help. And I wouldn't have had my child without hers.

Jeannine: I'm glad I know where my daughter is. A couple of weeks ago, I was walking down the street and I saw a child about her age. And it finally hit me that she was gone. I knew I had to see her one more time. So I made arrangements through the adoption agency and went to visit her with my mother. My daughter's so beautiful and seems so very happy. She's certainly well cared for, large house, nice nursery. The crib has this carousel of animals dangling above it. It plays music when it goes round. The adopting parents seemed to like our visit, but after a while it just got too much for everyone. I do want to see my baby again, but I don't want to interfere in their lives.

Carol: I wanted my child to be beautiful. Being beautiful makes life easier. Being beautiful makes life more beautiful. When I looked at Eva's photograph, tough times in Kosovo had creased lines between her brows and around her mouth. But Eva was beautiful. I know you think that I'm a cold woman for asking Eva to be my gestational carrier. I know you think that I have no right to a child, that it is my fault I waited too long, that I thought of my self, my career, rather than my child. That running out of eggs was some divine retribution for the career oriented life I led. But I really wanted to have a child. I go to sleep convincing myself that I have everything and I awake knowing I have nothing. Nothing now that my baby is gone to where she will have nothing. Well, nothing but love. I will never again risk breaking my heart over a broken surrogate contract. So my name languishes on long adoption lists. Lists of women like me who so want a child to love, a child to love them. Lists of women like me who know they will never have a child. Lists of modern women, cursed by the same thirst for a child that has parched women since Old Testament times. A tradition-taught thirst that makes women blind to their own beauty. We are sentenced from birth to one day address having a child. We may choose not to. We may want a child and not be able to. I am cursed by the knowledge that I could have had a child.

Stacey: I wish I knew where Eva went.

Jeannine: *[looks directly at the audience]*

I know. She went back to Kosovo.

[Jane begins singing, followed by Eva and other cast members.]

Savo Vodo hej lane

Sava River you are my lamb

Savo Vodo moj dragane

Sava River my dear friend

Savo Vodo pozdravi mi

Sava River please say hello for me

Dragog

To my loved one

FINIS

Acknowledgements

We would like to thank Rebecca Cann and Louise Fagan for their multiple contributions.

A Child on Her Mind was published in *Mother Life: Studies of Mothering Experience* Pedagon Publishing V. Bergum, J. Van Der Zalm (Eds.).[43]

---

[43] J. Nisker, V. Bergum, A Child on Her Mind, in V. Bergum, J. Van Der Zalm (eds.), *Mother Life: Studies of Mothering Experience*, Edmonton, AB: Pedagon Publishing, 2007, pp. 364-398.

Camouflage

with Kathy Tomanec

To generations of women,

To their children

To our children

Characters

Man, can be from age 30 to 50. He wears blue jeans and a casual shirt.
Camouflage Man, can be from age 30 to 50. He wears hunting camouflage pants and jacket.
Woman, can be from age 30 to 50. She wears either a cotton summer dress or blue jeans and a T-shirt.

Man: The violent winds that ripped the roads

And downed the power in paradise,

Queued campers and cottagers in an hour-long line

Before the general store's outdoor phone.

I stand next in line,

A respectable distance behind a thirty-something man

In green-brown hunting camouflage,

Yet close enough to prevent another

From butting in.

He puts his quarter in the slot,

Quickly looks over his shoulder at me,

And tells the operator,

Camouflage Man:

"Calling collect."

Woman:

I stand at the front of our house,

Looking out at the flowers.

My garden's a lovely place to be.

Even strangers coming to the door comment,

It's a lovely place to be.

Just last Saturday a delivery man,

With a "mother's boy" look to his face,

Said, "You have a beautiful garden."

I smiled at him and said, "Thank you."

As he walked away, he looked over his shoulder,

And bobbed, "The colours are wonderful."

I again smile, "Thank you."

Man: Even at my polite distance,

The post-storm calm makes it too easy to overhear

The man bravado to his wife,

How he had helped his fishing buddies

Defy the "once-in-a-century storm."

Just as it appears that the phone would be returned

To its Northern Bell receptacle,

The man matter-of-factly asks,

Camouflage Man:

"Did you go out?"

Man: A few seconds later,

His voice scantily dressing anger in nonchalance,

Camouflage Man:

> "You went to Denise's house?"

> "How did you get there?"

> "Linda picked you up?"

> "Who else was there?"

> "Are you sure no one else was there?"

Woman:

> The sun is hot on my face and legs.

> It feels good to be wearing shorts.

> A blue sky with puffs of white clouds

> Looks down on the house,

> And sees it's shaped like the letter H,

> With the openings of the H facing the front and back doors.

> Standing at either door,

> I am hugged by the flowers edging the walls,

> Pinks, blue, and white.

> The colours enter my eyes

> And live inside of me,

> Stored up,

> And are sent on bit by bit to my chest as needed.

Camouflage Man:

> "What time did you get home?"
>
> "Who drove you home?"
>
> "Are you sure you were home by then?"

Man: The politeness of his voice cannot conceal his rage.

        Yet his interrogation also reveals reticence,

        Even self-reprimand.

        This confuses me,

        And, I believe, confuses him.

Camouflage Man:

> "I'll be right home,"

Man: He says as he slams and stares at the phone.

        His hard hanging-up

        Surges through the stillness,

        But purges neither his anger nor bewilderment.

        His long staring at the phone

        Surfaces murmurs from the line behind me.

        The camouflage man looks over his shoulder

        To confront brown eyes too close to his blues:

        Studying his blues,

Staring helplessly at his blues

Conveying knowledge of him,

Conveying openness to conversation.

His eyelids tighten in question.

He turns his body to go.

I remain in his path,

Much longer than politeness permits.

Then silently allow him by.

I gently lift the phone,

Drop in my quarter

But cannot dial.

Instead I turn my head

And stare over my shoulder at the camouflage man,

Marching off with determination.

Again, murmurs from the long line.

I turn my head back to the phone,

And dial.

Woman:

Looking through patio doors at back,

I see the faucet and hose

I use every second day for watering.

Water drips on the bricks.

I let it drip.

It keeps the ground there moist

So Freddy the Frog will come around.

Freddy is large,

Almost the size of my fist,

Almost red,

Really a toad.

I talk to him while we water the flowers together.

Man: On every Friday of the 18 years

I lived in my wonderful childhood home

I remember seeing Eva.

Eva helped my mother dissolve the disorder

Three far too active and not-at-all responsible kids

Incurred on our house.

She came every Friday.

Of course we didn't appreciate Eva.

Far from it.

Eva was like a too-wise-to-us aunt,

Admonishing us each week

For our seeming lack of regard for the mother

Eva knew we dearly loved.

Eva would have admonished us more

If she knew my mother always cleaned the house thoroughly

The evening before the morning Eva came.

We saw Eva as my gentle mother's strong protector,

But rather than acknowledge her importance,

We teased her as children do.

She got us back by hiding our things,

Like my baseball bat or glove.

We were always too embarrassed to call her

To find out her hiding places.

Woman:

Four years ago winter came suddenly and stayed,

Turning my garden white and grey.

A small terry kitchen towel hung on the clothesline,

It had somehow escaped my final gathering.

It's faded yellow, orange, and red flowers

Moved gently in the breeze.

I've hung a towel out each winter since;

A single clothespin in one corner to allow maximum movement,

Just enough tether to be free.

What soul they show.

Straight through the harshest winters they hang in there:

Frolicking,

Spinning,

Sometimes even waltzing.

I always set the towel as far from the house as possible.

Just a bit away from the bushes,

So it won't get tangled.

Man: The last time I see Eva

Is at the cemetery after my mother's interment.

I am in my late twenties.

She her late forties I would guess,

About my mother's age.

The many mourners have lined out

Through the cemetery's black iron gates.

I trail behind,

Alone,

Not wanting to leave my mother.

When I walk out the gate, I see Eva,

Waiting.

She hesitantly greets me,

"I'm sorry Jeffrey, I'm sorry Jeffrey,"

Slowly and painfully.

I had not been called Jeffrey

Since my mother could speak.

That and the accent I had not heard

Since I lived in Toronto in my mother's house.

That and Eva's tears,

Immobilize me in our sorrow.

We hold each other without hugging.

Eva's eyes dart from mine,

Through the gate to my mother's grave.

I realize that she must not have been at my mother's graveside.

That Eva probably thinks entering the cemetery

Is reserved for family and friends,

And doesn't realize she is both.

Perhaps she believes the cemetery

Is for members of a particular religion.

I ask Eva if she wants to go to my mother's grave.

She shakes her head, "No."

I say, "I'll come with you,"

She shakes her head, "No."

I helplessly stare at her grief.

"Thanks for coming Eva," I say,

Before walking off toward the large black funeral car,

Not so patiently waiting for me.

Woman:

In the patio doors at back,

I can see my reflection,

But not clearly.

I look through the blurred image of my face

To see the flowers,

But I cannot see their colours.

They look grey.

I move closer to be able to see the colours.

But now I can't see my face at all;

I see my husband's face,

Looking over my shoulder,

Laughing at me.

But it can't really be his face.

He's away with his buddies.

Before he left,

He hid the keys to our second car as is his practice.

But I've made extra keys.

He also corrupted the engine lines,

Which I've learned to reattach,

And re-detach before he returns.

Man: Before entering the car,

I stare over my shoulder at Eva.

She has entered the cemetery

And is walking toward my mother's grave.

I am asked to enter the car but cannot.

I see Eva stand before the fresh earth,

Then drop to her knees at my mother's feet.

I am again asked to enter the car.

I comply and close the door.

I see Eva through the side window,

Lying face down in the fresh earth,

Arms extended,

Lying prostrate above my mother,

Hugging my mother.

As the funeral car pulls away,

I look over my shoulder at Eva.

She is lying perfectly still.

I do not demand the car stop,

So I can run back to console Eva.

I let it hurry away so we can receive the mourners

Accumulating at my parents' home.

Woman:

My face is wet, salty.

Something bumps me from behind.

I turn around quickly.

The wind is gently hushing through leaves and petals,

Coming in through the windows,

Cooling the tears on my face.

I turn to the glass door again.

There I am.

I see my eyes open wide.

I see my hand on my mouth.

My skin glistens.

I wrap my fingers around the door handle.

I count my fingers slowly.

One, two, three, four, five.

One, two, three, four, five.

One, two, three, four, five.

When I am finished counting,

I look in the glass again.

The flowers are there.

Man: Eva stopped her husband's abuse with a kitchen knife.

My father's long-distance words three years after my

mother's death,

"Eva killed her husband,"

Was my first clue to Eva's experience.

My father described Eva's many years of suffering,

Of tolerating the intolerable for her children's sake.

And when they went away to university,

How she defended against her abuse

By stabbing her abuser.

My self-centred childhood hurry had obviated inquiry

Of the muffled weeping in our kitchen,

That "shushed" and subsided

When I opened the door from school.

But not quite quickly enough for me not to perceive

Something was deeply upsetting Eva.

Woman:

The children are in bed now.

Tired from all their learning and doing of play.

I watch as waves of loss of consciousness wash over them.

Their mouths and hands gently twitch.

Eyes flutter.

As always, a smile quickly passes over the baby's face.

They are deep in sleep,

My guarded treasures.

The night has gotten heavy.

It is dark and a thick warm fog waits outside.

I lie in bed and stare into it through the big screened window.

I want the fog to come inside

And envelop me in its darkness.

I like these nights.

Sometimes I imagine hearing a foghorn

Calling from far away;

Sounding so earnest and insistent,

Like an elephant trumpeting,

A protector in the dark.

I lie on my back for a while,

Just for a change.

My body grows heavy.

My elephant calls again.

This time from farther away.

Man: My father was a character witness at Eva's trial.

I, of course, was not there:

Far too busy with patients and kids,

Too far away in emotion

To travel home for Eva.

Although the verdict prevented more prison for Eva,

The courtroom ordeal was more indignity endured

By a woman who had already endured

Society-ignored and thus society-sanctioned violation

For so many years.

Woman:

There is an alarm going off.

The alarm is in my chest.

Something is bumping me from behind.

Pushing at me.

I hear my elephant.

It is screaming.

I peer hard into the fog and follow the sound.

I cannot see my elephant but I know it is there.

Its screams cannot be buffered by the fog.

Man: My mother was the most compassionate woman I knew;

My father, the strongest man.

They would have done something about Eva's abuse if

they had known.

Or would they?

Or could they?

Eva had two children.

She may have wanted to protect them.

And if they could not help Eva,

Who could?

Recent immigrants have little social support,

And fear government-sponsored services.

Woman:

Oh there,

There's my elephant,

Standing on a little hill

That can hardly contain the four frantic stamping feet.

The legs bend and strain with each blast.

It's okay, my elephant.

It's okay.

Even though your purple-blue skin is hot and wet,

And your wide open eyes are red with blood,

And tears flow off your long lashes,

Even in this desperation, you have such a gentle face.

I want to hug you,

Calm you,

But you're so much bigger than I.

I hear someone screaming.

"The garden," I whisper.

"I can't see it!"

Man: I still stare over my shoulder at Eva,

Her face buried in the earth of my mother's grave;

Her lack of self-worth insisting

That "real" family members and friends leave

Before she can enter the cemetery.

I still stare over my shoulder at the camouflage man,

At the problem I allowed to walk away in paradise,

At the opportunity forever dissolved in the safety of silence.

What could have been lost through a kind conversation?

Did my Canadian politeness prevent privacy invasion?

Or was it a seminar at which "experts" cautioned clinicians

That unlike in "cases" of child abuse,

The "abused woman" must initiate the conversation,

"Must be ready" to seek help;

That unsolicited offers of help

Could harden the hurt,

That all we can do is leave pamphlets in waiting rooms,

Posters on walls,

Perhaps ask questions about bruises.

But when no bruises clue,

No conversation can occur.

Or can it?

I hope the "experts" are wrong,

Because I'm not sure I can be silent again.

FINIS

Acknowledgements

Portions of Camouflage were published in *Canadian Medical Association Journal*.[44]

---

[44] J.A. Nisker, A jury of my peers, *Canadian Medical Association Journal*, 1996, 155(6), 796.

Philip

To my children

Characters

Loudspeaker Voice
Philip, a 12-year-old boy.
Mother
Father
Nurse 1
Nurse 2
Nurse 3
Nurse 4
IV Nurse
Chemo Nurse, a woman in her forties or fifties.
Breakfast Server, a woman in her forties or fifties.
Vampire, a woman in her forties or fifties.
Fellow, a man.
Doctor, a man.

[A radio studio, with a large neon-like "ON AIR" sign hangs stage back above the simulated glass of the engineer's booth. At stage front, three microphone stands each hold a microphone with a round spit filter. Philip stands behind the microphone stage left, facing the audience. The other actors, whose voices become Philip's mother, father, nurses, doctors, and other hospital personnel, sit on chairs in a semicircle facing the audience stage centre, slightly back of the microphones until their lines approach. All actors hold the script in loose sheets of paper and will let each page fall when completed (rather than turning their pages). The large "ON AIR" sign turns red.]

Loudspeaker voice:

    Three, two, one.

Philip: I follow my parents through the atrium

    Of gift shops,

    Coffee shops,

    Fundraising banners,

    Helium-raising balloons.

    Balloons are everywhere,

    Even painted on the walls.

Mother: Everything will be fine this time, Philip.

    I just know it.

Philip: I follow my parents onto a balloon-assisted elevator.

    My father presses a button from my past.

Father: Here we go, Philip.

Philip: The elevator doors open

          To a too familiar floor,

          With more balloon-painted walls,

          And,

Nurse 1: [*quickly*]

          Lookin' good, Philip!

          Saw your name on admissions.

Nurse 2: [*quickly*]

          Great to see you again, Philip.

          Welcome back.

Nurse 3: [*quickly*]

          Even more freckles than last time, Philip.

          When was that?

Philip: About a year ago.

Nurse 3: That long?

Philip: Clearly I've been here before.

          Twice times before.

          I know too well its cheerer-uppers:

          Nurses,

Orderlies,

Candystripers.

Do you know why they're called candystripers?

Because they used to wear cotton-candy-pink-striped

uniforms.

But since I've been coming here,

They seem to wear various pastel-coloured smocks

Over their street clothes.

First time here, I had a huge crush

On Wednesday afternoon's candystriper.

Really cute.

She always wore a yellow smock

Over her T-shirt and blue jeans.

I looked forward all day Wednesdays to seeing her,

Until she finally came in after school.

At least I looked forward to seeing her until the amphotericin

started.

Then I didn't want to see her anymore.

Nurse 3: Just turn left and go down to the nurses' station, Philip.

I'm sure you remember where it is.

You remember everything.

264

Philip: In this get-well warren,

Even the vampires are cheery,

And there are many vampires here,

But different from movie vampires.

For example, they arise at dawn here,

Instead of disappearing into their caves or coffins;

They wear white or some pastel colour,

Never black;

And they're more interested in the veins in your arms

Than in your neck.

It must be hard for vampires to be cheery,

Having to puncture kids every morning

[Transylvanian accent]

Because they vant to take dare blood.

The young kids squirm and scream

Even before they're bitten.

But someone has to do their evil deeds,

So I'm nice to them.

When they say

[Transylvanian accent]

"Gut morning"

I respond,

[Transylvanian accent]

"You vant to bite my arm?

Gut vit me."

That makes the scared kids smile,

Because they know Count von Count from *Sesame Street.*

But my joking stops once amphotericin starts.

Nurse 4: Hey, Philip, my main man,

How old are you now?

Philip: Twelve.

Nurse 4: Twelve?

You sure you're twelve?

Last time you were here, we thought you were seventeen.

Just small for your age.

Philip: Only the doctors aren't always cheery here.

And their medical students and residents,

At least when my doctor's around.

When he's not, they joke around a bit:

Like last time one called me "Einstein,"

Another, "Motor Mouth."

266

But mostly they just hit on the nurses.

And after the amphotericin started,

I didn't feel like talking,

Let alone laughing,

So they left me alone.

Nurse 4: Follow me, Philip,

I'll get your chart.

I think you're in the same room as last time.

Philip: Last time,

I try not to think about last time,

I was here a month:

Submitting to nightly perfusions of promise,

That, in reality, were infusions of infirmity,

Sleep deprivation,

Amphoterrorism.

Nurse 4: Let me see, Philip,

Right,

Let's go.

Philip: It is the same room,

But not the same bed.

I try not to let my smile melt

In the fluorescent shadow of the IV tree

Growing from the head of the bed.

A tree that will soon dangle unforgiving fruit.

I sit on the edge of the bed.

My parents stand looking at me for a while,

Then at each other.

I do not challenge my mother's parting prognosis,

Mother: Everything will be fine this time, Philip.

I just know it will.

Philip: Or my father's,

Father: Remember how confident the doctor is

That the new anti-side-effect drug will work.

Philip: Their assurances are as much for them

As they are for me.

They know I'm reluctant to return to this place.

Reluctant to re-awaken its amphotericin nights.

Amphotericin is a cancer drug,

But I don't have cancer.

They also use it sometimes for what I have

To "ameliorate the symptoms."

Nurse 3: Just need to take your temperature, Philip.

Philip: I suck on the thermometer like a lollipop.

Nurse 3: Very funny, Philip.

          You know the drill.

Philip: I wobble it around in my mouth,

          Sort of like Joe Camel

          Smoking a Camel.

Nurse 3: C'mon, Philip

          Keep it still.

Philip: Last time I was here,

          Puking my guts out,

          One of the nurses said I was "an intrepid young man."

          I hate to admit it but I had to look "intrepid" up.

          Good word.

          Maybe my wanting to stay intrepid

          Is why I'm back.

          That and because of my parents.

          There's a beep.

          I hand the nurse her thermometer.

Nurse 3: Temperature's normal, Philip.

          Have a good night.

Philip: The ward quickly softens to sleep.

The kids in the three other beds

Nestle into their pillows.

They're probably much sicker than me.

Definitely much younger than me,

And have high sides on their beds caging them in.

They also have mobiles dangling above their heads:

Carousels of farm animals,

Zoo animals,

Birds.

The hospital somehow silences the musical mechanisms,

Or there would be a cacophony of tinkling tunes.

But a cacophony would be better than this silence of anticipation.

The IV nurse comes in

And heads straight to where veins should be

On the back of my left hand,

Stopping only briefly to "hang" a clear IV bag from the tree,

Containing the "normal saline" that will keep my "vein open,"

And to whisper,

IV Nurse:

[whispers]

Good evening, Philip.

Philip: She taps the back of my hand

To stand the veins up.

IV Nurse:

[whispers]

Nice to see you again, Philip.

Philip: Of course I think, "I wish I could say the same"

But say

[whispers]

"Nice to see you too."

IV Nurse:

[whispers]

Need to start your IV

So you can start your medicine.

Philip: *[whispers]*

I know.

She's still slapping the back of my left hand

I silently plead that a vein "comes up" and is very visible.

She stares at her chosen target.

The IV insertion hurts just as much as last time.

She smiles sympathetically.

She's having trouble "hitting" the vein

Just like last time.

IV Nurse:

[whispers]

Sorry, Philip.

Philip: She tries another vein.

I try to suppress sounds of pain.

She knows I know she's having trouble.

IV Nurse:

[whispers]

Almost got it, Philip.

Sorry.

I'll try your other hand.

Philip: She starts slapping the back of my right hand

They like putting IVs in hands

To allow the patient "greater mobility,"

Even though the veins are small.

IV Nurse:

Got it.

Philip: The nurse quickly tapes the IV to my hand,

And tells me to keep my wrist straight

Because "the IV's tempermental."

She tapes a plastic splint to the front of my wrist

To make sure I keep it straight.

Says,

IV Nurse:

[whispers]

That should do it, Philip.

Have a good night.

Philip: And leaves.

The salty fluid drips

Into the clear plastic reservoir

At the top of the IV

Premonisce what will come.

Too soon, another nurse comes in.

This one will "hang" the amphotericin.

She smiles encouragingly,

Chemo Nurse:

[whispers]

How's it going, Philip?

Philip: [*whispers*]

Fine, thank you.

First she "hangs" another clear bag.

This one contains potassium and other electrolytes

To replace those my body will barf

Into the aquamarine "k-basin"

Sitting ominously on the bedside table.

It's really called a kidney basin.

Because it's kidney-shaped.

The she swabs another of the "nipples" in my IV's tubing,

And plugs in the needle from the electrolyte bag.

Chemo Nurse:

[whispers]

Your IV's running well, Philip.

Philip: Her encouraging smile seems pasted on now,

As she "hangs" the Dijon mustard-coloured amphotericin,

Swabs another nipple,

And inserts its spear.

The poisonous mustardy drips stain the clear chamber,

Her encouraging smile continues

As she hangs an opaque white bag,

Which must contain the experimental drug

They hope will slay amphotericin's sins.

She swabs the final nipple,

And plugs hope in.

Then quickly adjusts the "drip rates."

Chemo Nurse:

[whispers]

Here we go, Philip.

See you tomorrow night.

Philip: She turns to go but stops.

She wiggles the big toe of my right foot and says,

Chemo Nurse:

Everything will be okay, Philip.

Philip: I try not to stare at the mustardy drips

As they slowly tick what will come.

I stare at the ceiling instead.

Hundreds of tiny black holes stare back

From greyish rectangular panels,

Hiding the wires and pipes and stuff.

One panel was removed last time,

And a man in orange overalls

Climbed up a ladder and shined a big square flashlight in.

The nurse had herded us out of the room,

But I watched from the doorway.

I stare harder at the holes.

Their pattern seems completely random.

I also see tiny lines in the panels.

I hadn't noticed them before.

They give the effect of elevation lines

On a topographical map.

I keep the words of the nurse that hung the side-effect drug

Echoing off the walls,

Chemo Nurse:

[whispers]

Everything will be okay, Philip.

Philip: She might have seen the drug successfully work.

She might know for certain that the new drug

Will make this "course" of amphotericin "tolerable."

"Course" is doctor talk for having to receive amphotericin

Every night for three weeks.

"Tolerable" is doctor talk for not puking my guts out

Every night for three weeks.

Chemo Nurse:

[whispers]

      Everything will be okay. Philip.

Philip: Maybe the milky-looking potion

      Will be magic after all.

Chemo Nurse:

[whispers]

      Everything will be okay, Philip.

Nurse 4: [*whispers*]

      Just making rounds.

      Everything okay, Philip?

Philip: [*whispers*]

      Yes, thank you.

      I wish I were still young enough

      To have a musical mobile,

      Cheer the air above my bed.

      Or even a non-musical mobile,

      Spaceships would be best,

      So I could dream of leaving.

      But instead I have IV bags

> Two clear,
>
> One white,
>
> One murky mustard.
>
> All void of melody and mirth.
>
> One bag filled with fear and foreboding.

Chemo Nurse:

> *[whispers]*
>
> Everything will be okay, Philip.

Philip: Midnight passes on the Timex Ironman

> My father gave me when I started high school last fall.
>
> I'm in a special program for kids like me.
>
> To make things more challenging.
>
> At least the novels are better.

Chemo Nurse:

[whispers]

> Everything will be okay, Philip.

Philip: At 2:15, the first ripples reach my core.

> Soon huge waves of ache
>
> Crash right through me,
>
> Cannonballing my supper

Into the kidney-shaped pool I precariously hold.

I try to contain the splash within its aquamarine rim,

But brownish green splatters the white bedsheets.

I try to mop it up with a facecloth between heaves.

Chemo Nurse:

[whispers]

Everything will be okay, Philip.

Philip: Maybe I should press the button for a nurse?

A nurse's hands could dim amphotericin for a while.

No, I'm too old for that.

And the nurses are very busy.

Only two of them on the ward at night

Due to the funding cutbacks.

Chemo Nurse:

[whispers]

Everything will be okay, Philip.

Philip: Only the white adhesive tape wrist shackle

Keeps me here.

That and my promise to my parents

To try again.

I barf again.

My k-basin's overflowing.

I press the button for a nurse.

Nurse 4: *[pauses, then whispers]*

Sorry, Philip.

Let me clean things up a bit.

You're doing fine.

Philip: She gives me another k-basin.

Nurse 4: I'll come back too.

Philip: The storm drags me to dawn.

I hear its cheery nurse chirpings

Of exaggerated good mornings.

There's nothing good about my morning.

Nothing will be good about my day.

I'll be too tired to open any of the books

My parents bought me as going-in presents.

I was really hoping to read *The Odyssey*,

Then A Prayer for Owen Meany,

Then The Life of Pi.

But then I was really hoping

The anti-side-effect drug would work.

Now my books' presence in my backpack

Just adds extra heaviness.

I try to lift my head

To greet the woman delivering breakfast,

But can't.

Breakfast Server:

[Spanish accent]

Breakfast.

Philip: She puts the tray on the over-the-bed table.

I work up a smile and am about to say "Nada"

When I see a vampire hovering over her shoulder,

I close my eyes in surrender.

Vampire:

[Transylvanian accent]

It von't hurt a bite.

Philip: She's right.

It hurts way more than "a bit"

After I put "pressure" on her puncture hole,

For almost the prescribed two minutes,

I decide to get out of bed

And try to start my day.

As I'm brushing my teeth,

I see my doctor enter the room,

His flowing white coat

Followed by a clothes line of white coats

Of the younger doctors and students.

They circle like swans around the bed nearest the door

across the room,

Stay for a few minutes

Then circle the bed beside it:

My doctor always going to the foot of the bed,

The "fellow" presenting the "case" to the head of the bed,

Then the cygnets circle quickly, forming around the bed.

("Fellows" can be women doctors, too

But this one's a man.)

Knowing the drill, I return to my bed

Before they flock around it.

I wouldn't want to slow them down.

Fellow: This 12-year-old boy was admitted yesterday for amphotericin.

His preadmission blood work indicated we could start treatment.

He—

Doctor: [*interrupts*]

Philip, I heard you were admitted yesterday,

How have you been?

Philip: Fine, Doc.

Fellow: I wrote his medication orders yesterday morning,

So he should have had his first dose of amphotericin last night.

Yes, I see the bag is still hanging.

Philip: Everyone stares over my head

At the empty mustard-tinged bag

Except my doctor and me.

I actually make a point of not looking at the bag,

Until a nurse comes and disposes of the wretched thing.

To the hospital's incinerator, I hope.

Or at least to a dump with the hospital's radioactive stuff,

And its toxic chemical waste.

My doctor looks at me sympathetically.

Doctor: How did you manage last night, Philip?

Philip: I can handle it, Doc.

My doctor turns to his learners.

From Calcedonies to Orchids

Doctor: In addition to amphotericin,

Philip is receiving an experimental drug

To ameliorate its side effects.

It has had very promising results.

In clinical trials with cancer patients.

Philip: They all nod very interested.

My doctor explains that because I don't have cancer,

He was fortunate to get the drug for me "off trial."

They all nod again.

A cygnet asks a biochemistry question

To impress my doctor.

It works.

My doctor beams and fires off a mini lecture,

Also in biochemistry language,

On the theory of how the side-effect drug works.

Unless my barfing woke up the other kids

I'm the only one in the room who knows it doesn't work.

Doctor: Any other questions?

Philip: Necks bowing, the white circle dissipates,

Then reforms around the bed beside me.

I silently repeat "I can handle it" over and over

Until my doctor leads the white coats out of the room.

Then I whisper, "I don't think I can handle it."

Nurse 2: Here let me get rid of these, Philip.

Philip: The nurse takes the IV bags away.

My body has lost the strength I summoned for my doctor,

And my head collapses on the pillow.

In an hour or so, I hear the breakfast server coming back.

I hear her removing my tray,

Then putting it back.

Breakfast Server:

[Spanish accent]

You must eat,

Philip: She pauses,

Breakfast Server:

[Spanish accent]

Felipe.

Philip: She must have looked at the name card at the foot of my bed.

Breakfast Server:

[Spanish accent]

You must eat to get well, Felipe.

Philip: I lift my head long enough to say in *Sesame Street* Spanish,

"Gracias, no tengo hambre, Senõra."

Breakfast Server:

[excitedly]

Hablas Espanol, Felipe?

Philip: Nada.

Breakfast Server:

[Spanish accent]

Muy bien

Veo, tu peudes hablas un poquito de Espanol

Por favor, come algo

Tienes que mantenerte fuerte.

Philip: I open my eyes.

She has walked to the head of my bed

And is staring into my eyes,

Breakfast Server:

[Spanish accent]

Por favor, to eat, try.

Philip: And leaves.

I try to go back to sleep but can't.

The hospital noises are amplified when you're tired.

I get out of bed and aimlessly wander the halls.

The kids on the floor are sicker than me.

I try not to meet anyone's eyes

Because I don't have the energy to smile,

Let alone have a conversation.

A nurse comes right up to me.

I avoid her eyes,

But she touches my shoulder and asks,

Nurse 3: Do you want to go to the craft room, Philip?

Philip: No, thank you.

Nurse 3: What about the book cart?

Philip: No, thank you,

I've brought several books from home.

She smiles and goes down the hall.

I return to my room to try to read,

But can't.

Then I try to draw with similar results.

I don't even attempt to write.

Too soon it's "visitors' hours,"

And I have to hide last night from my mother

When she comes in looking worried and asks,

Mother: How did it go, Philip?

Philip: And from my father,

Father: Did the new medication work?

Philip: But I know they know it didn't work,

Because I see them surreptitiously staring

At the dark circles disguising my eyes.

But they can't admit they know.

For that would admit they know

What I will go through tonight.

I don't have much to say,

Which of course is unusual for me,

And of course worries them.

They find my quietude uncomfortable,

So I try to make conversation.

They can't stay long anyway.

They both took the afternoon off work to come down here.

It's a two-hour drive.

So when my father squeezes my mother's arm,

And says,

288

Father: We have to go, son.

Philip: And stands,

      And my mother says,

Mother: We love you, Philip.

Philip: I'm almost happy to see them go.

      The grey brick outside the window is reddening

      I hope the reddening will last a long time

      Holding off,

Loudspeaker voice:

      Visiting hours are now over.

Philip: I hide last night from the chemo nurse,

      As she hangs tonight's amphotericin,

      And the way overrated side-effect medicine,

      And says,

Chemo Nurse:

[whispers]

      Good night, Philip.

Philip: I hide last night from myself

      Until the first amphotericin aggressions

Writhe my courage.

I am still awake in the morning

When the white flotilla flocks my bed.

I'm determined to hide the new last night from my doctor

But when he asks directly,

Doctor: How was last night, Philip?

Philip: I weaken,

"Actually, not so hot, Doc."

Doctor: You can handle it, Philip.

Philip: I think, "No I can't,"

But say,

"Doc, isn't there an alternative to amphotericin?

I mean it's not like I have cancer."

He looks at me sympathetically, for what seems to be a long time.

Doctor: No son,

You don't have cancer.

Philip: Then let me try something else.

Doctor: I'm sorry, Philip.

I wish there was something else.

Philip: Then maybe less amphotericin.

Doctor: I'm sorry, it won't work then.

Philip: That's okay, Doc.

Just thought I'd ask.

Doctor: See you tomorrow, Philip.

Philip: This day seems longer.

Probably because I'm too tired

To push my IV tree around.

My parents eventually come in,

After pausing to press their smile buttons

Just outside the door.

Mother: Hello, my young man.

Father: I see you're keeping your chin up, Philip.

Philip: I feel like saying,

That's because I pressed my smile button too.

But of I course don't.

There's no point.

"I'm okay."

This will be the last time my parents visit until the weekend.

They can't keep taking afternoons off work,

And the long drive is just too much.

I try to keep smiling but can't.

So I tell them, "I want to try to sleep for a bit."

Mother: We'll watch you then.

Philip: I appreciate you coming all this way to see me.

But why don't you get an early start home.

It's okay.

Father: We'll get a coffee and come back later.

Philip: Too soon, they come back.

Too soon, it's—

Loudspeaker voice:

Visiting hours are now over.

Philip: Too soon, the amphotericin nurse comes in.

She's thinking about changing my IV.

Fortunately she decides the original will last a little longer.

Chemo Nurse:

I know it's tough on you, Philip.

Is there anything I can do?

Philip: I think, "Yes, there're three things:

First, don't plug your poison into me,

Second, say goodbye

And third, never come back,"

But say, "No thank you."

She plugs the poison in.

Chemo Nurse:

Good night, Philip.

Philip: This night seems longer.

I know I must accept my amphotericin-alloyed future,

But as the amphotericin bag drips its venom through my being,

And the anti-side-effect bag drips incompetence beside it,

And runnels of salt water drip into my mouth,

I change my mind.

I don't have to accept this.

Suddenly I feel better,

As if the experimental anti-side-effect infusion is actually working.

Of course it's not working at all,

But I giddily accept the amphotericin

And the wretchedness it wrecks upon me.

I even taunt the amphotericin bag:

"Hurt me tonight if you want,

Because it's your last chance.

Tomorrow I will refuse you.

Tomorrow night I will sleep.

The next day I will read again,

I will draw pictures again,

I will smile again,

I will be Philip again."

I spend the last hours till dawn

Rehearsing my refusal of amphotericin.

My dress rehearsal occurs

As the white coats tighten around the first

Then the second bed across the room.

Then my bed.

My doctor says,

Doctor: How did it go last night, Philip?

Philip: I inhale slowly,

Nod twice,

Exhale,

"Doc, I had my last ampho-terrible night."

FINIS

Acknowledgements

Portions of Philip were published in *Canadian Medical Association Journal*.[45]

[45] J. Nisker, Philip, *Canadian Medical Association Journal*, 2003, 168(6), 746-747.

Orchids

To those physically or cognitively different from "ideal"

"Everyone carries within themselves the whole condition of humanity ...."

Michel de Montaigne

"This is the stuff that dreams are made of ....."

Dashiell Hammett, *The Maltese Falcon*
from Shakespeare's *The Tempest*

"I know a place where dreams are born ....."

Betty Comden, Adolph Green, and Jule Styne, "Never
Never Land"
from the musical adaptation of J.M. Barrie's *Peter Pan*

Characters

Eight laboratory technicians.
Heather, a woman in her early thirties.
Rose, a woman in her early thirties.
Dr. Blume, a man in his forties or fifties.
Dr. Staiman, a man in his forties or fifties.

Scene 1

[The lights go up to display an assembly line of an unusual kind: a long laboratory bench, composed of eight technician stations, each with a large microscope bookended by test-tube trays, pipettes, and Petri dishes of exaggerated size. Eight laboratory technicians in flowing white lab coats intently gaze down their microscopes at the embryos they manipulate. Each tech is adorned in sterile garb—gloves, hats, masks, all white. In synchrony, they lift their heads from the microscope, turn right, turn left, pass the Petri dish to the next tech, then embrace the microscope's eyepiece again. The lab techs represent the well-motivated but often uncritical thinking of medical science. At the end of the song, a scrim curtain descends in front of the lab set, which remains in the background throughout the play.]

Song: Embryo Engineers

Verse 1: We are good lifeguards

Care for our kids

Help them swim

Lives begin

Beneath glass lids

Verse 2: We take our jobs

Seriously

Tiny hopes

Float

Precariously

From Calcedonies to Orchids

Chorus: Science blessed

Happiness

Proud to be

Embryo engineers

Verse 3: Trained to be cogs   We engineer

In this machine   We re-design

Holding hopes   What nature made

In microscopes   We can refine

Fulfilling dreams

Verse 4: We analyse   We make solutions   Science Reason

And then dissect   Help them survive   Calculation

Pour emotions   We study traits   Science Reason

In perfect potions   And then select   All

To help them thrive   To help them thrive   To help them thrive

Chorus: Science blessed

Happiness

Born to be

Embryo engineers

Science blessed

Happiness

Born to be

Embryo engineers

Embryo engineers

Scene 2

[At centre stage is a waiting room with four chairs. Rose is seated at stage left and Heather is seated at stage right. Two chairs in the middle separate them. All chairs are identical. Behind them hang four large pictures: Picasso's "Maternité," a large photograph of an orchid, a large picture with the letters L-O-V-E created out of a single baby picture reproduced multiple times, and a large picture of an orchid similarly created out of a computer-cloned baby picture. The table in front of the chairs bears Cosmopolitan and Chatelaine magazines and literature from the Infertility Awareness Association. Rose and Heather leaf through magazines, carefully respecting each other's space and privacy. Heather catches Rose's glance.]

Heather: Isn't this picture beautiful?

Rose: Yes, a perfect orchid. Did you know that orchid cultivators

manipulate the petals to look like our ...

[hesitates]

Heather: Our?

Rose: You know, the female ... our...

Heather: Our hoo-hahs?

Rose: They're genetically manipulating the blooms to be larger and

larger. I read somewhere that some flowers become so big

that they fall over on their stems.

Heather: [*laughs*]

Like tom turkeys.

Rose: Turkeys?

Heather: They've engineered male turkeys to have huge chests for extra white meat. But the toms keep falling over forward—they can't walk—and of course, they can't mate to pass on the genes for the extra white meat.

[laughs]

Rose:　No.

Heather: Divine retribution for crossing Mother Nature.

Rose:　Do you know that they've very successfully used genetics to breed *cattle* with more meat.

Heather: Red or white?

Rose:　I would guess red, for now anyway. My name's Rose.

[They shake hands.]

Heather: Heather.

Heather: How do they do it?

Rose:　Do what?

Heather: The cows!

Rose:　Oh! They take semen from bulls with genes for lots of meat, and inject it in the wombs of thousands of cows that also have genes for extra meat.

Heather: You're kidding!

Rose: It doesn't end there. They then take the embryos out of the genetically good cows and implant them in the wombs of less valuable cows, who then give birth to good-gene calves.

Heather: Why do they take them out?

Rose: Because the breeders don't want to risk losing the valuable cows during pregnancy or birthing.

Heather: Sort of a bovine *Handmaid's Tale*.

[pauses]

Anyway, do you live on a farm?

Rose: Are you kidding? No, I heard it on the CBC. Did you notice he name under that orchid?

Heather: Catalina staimanlina.

Rose: It was bred by Dr. Staiman, one of the doctors here.

Heather: A doctor that not only stops and smells the flowers but tries to make them —

[Rose and Heather speak simultaneously.]

... beautiful.

Rose: ... perfect.

[Rose and Heather laugh.]

Rose: I met Dr. Blume my last time here. I like him. He takes time to explain things.

Heather: I saw the IVF video when I got here this morning.

Rose: It's amazing what medical technology can do now. The ability of that ultrasound machine to look right inside you, to see your ovaries, and to guide that long needle that retrieves your eggs.

Heather: Wasn't that woman brave to be videoed?

Rose: I could never do that.

Heather: I especially liked the view through the microscope camera.
          Seeing embryos only a few cells old.

Rose: Which doctor are you seeing today?

Heather: I'm not sure. I understand they work as a team.

Scene 3

[Two focal points are illuminated on the stage to stage right and left of Rose and Heather. At stage left, Dr. Blume stands behind a lectern and behind him hangs a picture of a caduceus. This image is mirrored at stage right by Dr. Staiman, who stands behind a similar lectern, and behind him hangs a large picture of an orchid, above which is a banner that reads "The 12th Annual International Orchid Society Convention." Before the doctors begin their respective lectures (Dr. Blume to a medical school class, and Dr. Staiman to the orchid enthusiasts), the house lights are raised so the audience members feel they are alternatively medical students or members of the International Orchid Society, respectively.]

Dr. Blume:

> Good morning, class. Dr. Staiman was supposed to give this lecture but, and I am proud to say, is at this moment receiving a lifetime achievement award for his contribution to orchid genetics. He sends his apologies and says he will join us as soon as he can. Although Dr. Staiman and I practise medicine and do research together, he can engage you in genetic science much better than I. But I'll try my best.

Dr. Staiman:

> Good morning cultivators and thank you.

[cradles plaque]

> I am deeply honoured by this award. Genetic science allows us to create more beautiful orchids every year. Soon we will create perfect orchids.

Dr. Blume:

> Before we talk about genetic science, I want to take a moment to tell you that you already possess the brains, the heart, and the courage to become great doctors, and, just like the Scarecrow, the Tin Man, and the Lion, you don't need the great and powerful Oz—or the Dean—to bestow on you a diploma to give you what you already possess. The Tin Man travels to Oz for the heart he thought he lacked. But remember how, on the yellow brick road, he cradled Dorothy in caring arms and rusty tears. Being a compassionate individual, he craved the ability to care more. You're all caring individuals, or you would not have chosen this career. So, keep on like the Tin Man. Never allow the compassion that led you into medicine to dissolve in miles of medical ink and consuming call schedules.

Dr. Staiman:

> It's really not fair for me to accept this generous cheque that goes with this award.

[indicates plaque]

> You see, I get paid quite well for creating beautiful humans. And of course, there are many similarities between orchids

and humans, from the Greek word *orchid* having been bestowed on our special flower because of the resemblance of its root to a human testicle, to our work in genetically manipulating the orchid's central petal to resemble a woman's...well...as we medical types call them, labia. This work has helped medical science understand human genetic potential.

Dr. Blume:

In a perfect world, exploration of the ethical and social implications of genetic science should precede research and applications. In a perfect curriculum, ethics and social exploration should precede teaching scientific principles and clinical applications.

Dr. Staiman:

There are no constraints on how we can use genetic science to enhance orchids: DNA transfer, gene splicing, cloning.

Dr. Blume:

I must point out that without careful constraints, the rapid pace of genetic science and its new enhancement applications may be harmful to many. But the medical school curriculum insists that we start each subject area with scientific principles. So we will have to wait to explore the ethical and social implications of genetic science until this afternoon.

[PowerPoint slide of in vitro fertilization appears.]

Okay. Let's start at the beginning. Fertilization. Let's use *in vitro* fertilization to illustrate. In IVF, a woman receives fertility drugs to hyper stimulate her ovaries to create multiple eggs. These drugs may cause nausea, abdominal bloating. and pain. We then retrieve the eggs through transvaginal ultrasound-guided surgery. This is a very uncomfortable painful procedure but it has a much better pregnancy rate and is much safer than previous surgical strategies. The eggs are put in a Petri dish to which her partner's sperm is added and hopefully fertilization occurs. We then transfer up to three embryos to the woman's uterus and freeze the rest to transfer later in hopes that she won't have to go through the drugs and surgery again. The one-cell human embryo has inherited 23 chromosomes from its mother's egg and 23 chromosomes from its father's sperm. Within the chromosomes are the genes that help code our physical traits.

Dr. Staiman:

> We should applaud how the increasing capacity of genetic science combined with new fertilization technologies enhances our lives today in so many ways: not just in creating magnificent orchids, but the huge enetically modified strawberries and tomatoes we enjoy in all their glory. Orchid genetic science may one day not only help us feed the world by making crops resistant to parasites but may make people stronger and resistant to diseases. Soon, we will be able to enhance orchids to perfection. Soon, we will be able to insert genes directly into orchid seeds so generation after generation will possess all the traits we desire. Soon we will be able to construct any genetic code we want.

[Lab techs enter and form an arc behind Dr. Staiman. They wear mantles that transform their lab coats into gospel robes. Behind the doctors and in front of the scrim curtain, stained glass windows drop down and are backlit.]

Song: I Orchestrate My Orchids' Shape

Dr. Staiman:

> I orchestrate my orchids' shape

Techs: *[in gospel harmony]*

> Gene by gene

> Generation by generation

Dr. Staiman:

> I cultivate for beauty's sake

Techs: Dream by dream

> Celebration . Oh celebration

Dr. Staiman:

> I permutate to promulgate

Techs: Glean by glean

> Celebrate what we create

> Oh celebrate

Staiman and Techs:

> I orchestrate my orchids' shape

> Gene by gene

> Generation by generation

> I orchestrate my orchids' shape

> Celebrate

> What we create

> OH celebrate

> I cultivate for beauty's sake

> Dream by dream

> Each selection

I cultivate for beauty's sake

Celebrate

What we create

OH celebrate

I anticipate

Each deviate

Screen by screen

Rejection upon rejection

I anticipate each deviate

Celebrate

What we create

OH celebrate

Dr. Staiman:

Let's meditate

Techs: *[as a gospel response]*

Let's meditate

Dr. Staiman:

On my motivate

Techs: On his motivate

Dr. Staiman:

> I navigate
>
> The ameliorate
>
> Of genetic fate
>
> I castigate

Techs: He castigates

Dr. Staiman:

> And gene ablate

Techs: And gene ablate

Dr. Staiman: I aggregate	Techs: Aggregate
I insinuate	Insinuate
Til I fabricate	Fabricate
The transfigurate	The transfigurate
And celebrate	And celebrate

Dr. Staiman:

> Celebrate

Techs: Celebrate

Dr. Staiman:

> Not initiate

315

Techs: He won't initiate

Dr. Staiman:

> A syndicate

Techs: No syndicate

Dr. Staiman:

> Don't let me pontificate

Staiman and Techs:

[in exaggerated gospel harmony]

> I permutate to propagate
>
> Gene by gene
>
> Selection upon selection
>
> I permutate to propagate
>
> Celebrate
>
> What we create
>
> OH celebrate
>
> Celebrate
>
> What we create
>
> Oh celebrate
>
> Celebrate
>
> What we create
>
> Oh celebrate

Scene 4

[Spot on Heather and Rose in the waiting room. They smile at each other.]

Heather: There certainly are a lot of baby pictures in this room.

Rose: I suppose they're here to inspire positive thinking.

Heather: I stared at that "LOVE" one for quite a while before you

arrived. Do you realize it's created from thousands of tiny

identical baby faces?

Rose: So is the other orchid picture. Do you like them?

Heather: Well. There's something… uncomfortable about them …

Rose: Be careful, Heather. They're both my creations.

Heather: I'm sorry. We've just met and I've already managed to offend

you. I really am sorry.

[pauses]

If it helps, I know nothing about art.

Rose: I've been told my work is disconcerting. One baby picture

cloned over and over again is not what most people expect in

a picture.

Heather: They're quite remarkable.

Rose: Thank you. I actually got the idea from the Ancient Celts. At least from a book about them in art school. They carved identical patterns, varying only in size, on blocks of wood, dipped them in animal blood or vegetable dyes, and patiently stamped them over and over again on animal skins. The density difference between the larger and smaller images created the pictures. My computer can now create in a few hours what it took the Celts years to achieve. Fortunately they didn't patent the process.

Heather: How did the Celts come to have their art form displayed here?

Rose: The Clinic's administrator called me a few months ago to see if I could create some art in my signature style for this waiting room. I came here, looked at the space, presented a couple of concepts she liked and a month ago I delivered these.

Heather: What a beautiful baby. It must be hard to take baby portraits.

Rose: It is hard. Babies cry, frown, poop. But actually I don't take the pictures—I have an assistant. And even though every now and then her camera captures a perfect baby smile, I computer-modify each smile to give parents what they want—and pay me for.

318

Heather: I work with computers, too.

Rose: Really? What do you do?

Heather: I have a small computer software company.

Rose: Wonderful. How did you start it?

Heather: It took a while: um … early twenties training, late twenties writing endless computer codes through endless nights to prove myself to my boss — and me. Eventually I thought, "I can run my own business."

Rose: Are you on your own or do you have assistants?

Heather: At first I was on my own. I actually liked working alone. It was safer for me.

[quickly adds]

I mean for my business. But when my business grew I had to recruit help. And I was very lucky — I have some great programmers working with me.

Rose: You must have offered them something good — like more money.

Heather: I think my team joined me because they respected my talent. I think they stay — despite my quirks — because I respect their talent. Sean, of course, stays because he loves me.

Rose: Your husband?

Heather: And my best buddy. How did you meet your husband?

Rose: Alan spotted me in the university library. I was trying to reproduce a da Vinci body dissection. He fabricated an interest in art long enough to ask me out. I'm glad he did. What's Sean like?

Heather: People see Sean as your classic computer nerd. But if you take the time to listen to him, you can hear Sean's sensitivity, his love. Life is good. What's Alan like?

Rose: As he tells everyone, Alan has it all: great DNA and me.

Heather: DNA?

Rose: You know, genes for athleticism and the great body that goes with it — which is how he thinks he got me.

Heather: I'm sure there's more to Alan than DNA.

Rose: Of course. But Alan's life *was* preordained: university, marriage, well-paying job, big house, couple of cars, couple of charming children.

[pauses]

It's the charming children part that, as you must suspect, brings me here.

Heather: Yes. It was easier for me to start my business than start my baby.

Rose: If you don't mind my asking, why do you need IVF?

Heather: Damaged fallopian tubes.

Rose: I'm sorry. How did that happen?

Heather: I was pregnant five years ago and the embryo got stuck in my left tube. It ruptured and I almost bled to death. They had to do emergency surgery and remove the tube to stop the bleeding.

Rose: I'm so sorry.

Heather: It turned out that my other tube is also terribly scarred. So I could easily have another ectopic pregnancy. IVF is my safest and best chance of having a child.

Rose: Absolutely.

Heather: We're going to have to struggle to pay for it, but it's better than risking another ectopic pregnancy, or accepting not having a child.

Rose: For me, the price is definitely worth it.

Heather: Why can't you have children?

Rose: Actually, I can have children.

Heather: [*pauses*]

Then why—I'm sorry— I thought IVF was for infertility. I don't understand why you're here.

Rose:　There's a new method of genetic testing that uses IVF. It's called preimplantation genetic diagnosis.

Heather: Preimpl ... ?

Rose:　I know, it's a mouthful. They call it PGD for short.

Heather: I've never heard of it.

Rose:　It's a great scientific advance. They test your embryos before you're pregnant to make sure you only have normal embryos implanted in your uterus.

Heather: [*masks tics*]

"Normal embryos?" I don't understand.

Rose:　Remember the IVF videos?

Scene 5

[Dr. Staiman walks into Dr. Blume's spot and sits in chair next to the podium, and nods to Dr. Blume as he sits down. Dr. Blume returns the nod, then turns to his class.]

Dr. Blume:

> Here he is now. Class, I would like to introduce my colleague and friend, Dr. Staiman. He is respected equally for his work in both orchid and human genetics.

[Staiman approaches the podium and shakes Blume's hand.]

Dr. Staiman:

> Actually, I am much more respected for my work in orchid genetics than I am for my work in human genetics, as I hold 34 patents for orchid gene sequences, but alas only two human patents.

Dr. Blume:

> Dr. Staiman is being modest. He was the physician who helped perfect preimplantation genetic diagnosis, so I can think of no one better to explain it to you.

Dr. Staiman:

> But it was Dr. Blume's imagination that allowed those experiments to proceed, not to mention his skill in attracting research funding. I just translated it to biological reality.

Now my friend's imagination gives him nightmares, while I
sleep like a baby in sweet dreams of science.

Dr. Blume:

Tell them when your sweet dreams began.

Dr. Staiman:

I was 15 years old and was reading *Flowers for Algernon.*

Dr. Blume:

You may have seen the film adaptation, *Charly*, with Cliff
Robertson and Claire Bloom?

Dr. Staiman:

Any relation?

Dr. Blume:

Sorry.

Dr. Staiman:

Pity.

Dr. Blume:

Students, you will know Cliff Robertson as Spider-Man's
Uncle Ben. He was much younger when he won the Oscar
for Charly.

Dr. Staiman:

> Anyway, these great scientists developed a brain enhancing chemical that made this mouse, Algernon, a very smart mouse. So they approached this cognitively impaired man, Charly, to volunteer to be a human guinea pig.

Dr. Blume:

> Actually a human mouse.

Dr. Staiman:

> Anyway, Charly received the drug and he became a genius.

Dr. Blume:

> Tell them what happened at the end of the story.

Dr. Staiman:

> Well, the drug's effect proved to be short-lived and Charly slid back to his previous IQ of 60.

Dr. Blume:

> Sounds like a horror story.

Dr. Staiman:

> Just the opposite, class. It stimulated a certain 15-year-old whiz kid to dream that one day he could invent ways to develop superior intelligence.

Dr. Blume:

> Class, I saw Charly's story as a cautionary tale of the dangers of science proceeding without prior moral exploration —

[Dr. Staiman starts to talk but changes his mind.]

Dr. Blume:

> But as we both have patients to see soon, I will step back so Dr. Staiman can focus on scientific principles.

[Dr. Blume moves away to exit but stops.]

Dr. Staiman:

> And I'm sure, Dr. Blume, you would prefer them to learn in human not horticultural terms.

Dr. Blume:

> Or even mouse terms.

Dr Staiman:

> Okay ... so here we go. Preimplantation genetic diagnosis.

[PowerPoint presentation on PGD appears. An embryo biopsy film starts on the screen behind the podium.]

> We test the eight-cell embryo for genetic disease by removing a blastomere. Here the "holding pipette" embraces

the embryo with suction to keep it still. Either a dissolving solution or a laser opens a hole in the embryo and a blastomere is teased out. We extract the DNA and multiply it thousands of times to determine whether it carries *bad* genes. Only the embryos whose genetic markers are normal are transferred into the woman's uterus. The embryos with the bad genes are transferred to the stem cell lab. This year there are approximately 350 diseases that we can test for. Next year there will be many more.

[Dr. Blume takes a step back to the podium but stops and hangs his head.]

Dr. Blume worries about PGD and I see he's just itching to worry you.

Scene 6

[Spot on Heather and Rose in the waiting room.]

Heather: [*masking manoeuvres*]

> Is it the same type of IVF as for infertility?

Rose: It's exactly the same: same drugs, same ultrasounds, same egg
        retrieval surgery. We may even be here on the same
        days. We might become good friends. I understand that
        happens when women go through IVF together.

Heather: [*masking manoeuvres*]

> How did you find out about PGD?

Rose: When I came here to drop off the proofs of these pictures at
        the administrator's office, I noticed that the Clinic had
        changed its name from The Reproductive Medicine Clinic to
        The Reproductive and *Genetic* Technology Clinic. I asked
        her if the Clinic had a way to help me avoid having a child
        with a genetic disease. She said "We surely do," and
        introduced me to Dr. Blume.

Heather: [*Heather's masking manoeuvres gradually become more
        exaggerated.*]

> What do they do with the embryos that aren't completely
> "normal"?

Rose: Dr. Blume told me they used to discard them, but now, if I want to, I can donate them to research. I've already signed the consent form to donate mine to stem cell research.

Heather: Stem cell?

Rose: Perhaps my abnormal embryos will be developed into spinal cord cells to help quadriplegics lead more productive lives. Wouldn't that be amazing?

Heather: Rose,

[masking manoeuvres]

it seems like you're going through quite a lot when

[masking tics]

you could have a baby naturally.

Rose: I know it seems that way but...I was also pregnant once. I didn't have an ectopic like you but my pregnancy so was also a horrible experience.

Heather: What happened?

Rose: I had genetic testing done the usual way with amniocentesis. I had to wait until I was 16 weeks pregnant for there to be enough fluid for the doctors to take some safely. Then for the next two weeks I spent every minute hoping that my baby would be all right. But then the doctors told me that the fetus carried a marker for the genetic disease that runs in my family, I mourned from that moment on. While I was waiting the week for the procedure I felt the fetus move, and move, and move. Each movement made it that much harder.

Heather: I'm so sorry, Rose.

Rose: I was about halfway through my pregnancy when they injected the solution to try to kill the fetus and induce labour. I went through contractions, pain, waiting for the pain—it was horrible. I was terrified the baby would be born alive. I had been told that happens sometimes.

[pauses]

Anyway, having genetic testing done before my embryos are implanted means I will never have to go through that experience again. And I will be able to make sure that my baby doesn't have the disease that made my twin brother's life miserable.

Heather: [*masking manoeuvres*]

You have a twin brother?

Rose: Richard. He was hard to control and his outbursts were always getting him into trouble. I can't tell you how often my Dad had to go to the principal's office and take him home.

Heather: Hmm.

Rose: And the kids were always picking on him, you know, hitting him in the face with snowballs or mud just to see how crazy he would go. And he would go crazy, and that would get him into more trouble.

Heather: It's too bad he was picked on.

Rose: Well, he had these weird tics that made him swear and do other crazy things.

[Heather's face darkens quietly and her tics become accentuated.]

I was known as crazy Richard's sister and also teased mercilessly.

Heather: *[masking manoeuvres]*

I'm sorry.

Rose: Richard's disease really made life hell for all of us. My poor parents. We couldn't ever go to a restaurant

[Heather stands and walks a few steps forward.]

331

or Disney World, or any normal family thing. They were always afraid that Richard would disrupt everything and embarrass us.

[Heather's agitation increases, with tics. Rose pauses, something disturbs her. Heather paces, tics increase.]

Do you know about Tourette Syndrome?

Heather: [*tics*]

Yes.

[Heather has difficulty controlling her tics. Rose realizes that Heather has Tourette's.]

Rose: I'm sorry—I should have clued in from some of your movements. Uh... um... it was so insensitive of me... uh... I'm sorry.

Heather: [*tics*]

There's nothing to be sorry for.

[tics, loses control]

It's okay.

Rose: I can see that it's not okay.

Heather: I'm fine. I can control the tics. Just give me a minute.

[Heather tics. Music starts for song "Intensity."]

Rose: I bet most people don't realize that there's anything wrong
       with you. I didn't and my brother has Tourette's. You have
       such great control of yourself.

Song: Intensity

Heather:

Verse 1 I've worked hard to subdue this intensity inside me
         Trained my tics to maintain my poise
         I've learned to channel my energy
         But I still crave symmetry to quiet the noise

Verse 2 My tics don't harm anyone, even when they erupt
         And cause alarm in inquiring eyes
         I've learned to convert them so I don't disrupt
         The perfect pictures people seem to prize

Chorus   I have intensity that's hard to control
         A powerful propellant beneath my skin
         But I've learned strategies to help me hold
         Till I tamed my tension within

Verse 3 I suppress my compulsions so I appear calm
         Then my existence will not impose on anyone
         I found a way to belong
         I found the confidence to be strong

333

Chorus I have intensity that's hard to control

A powerful propellant beneath my skin

But I've learned strategies to help me hold

Till I tamed my tension within

Refrain I try controlling my intensity, but I love my life

It's hard controlling my intensity, but I love my life

I am controlling my intensity

Scene 7

[Spots on Dr. Blume and Dr. Staiman standing at the lectern.]

Dr. Blume:

> Dr. Staiman and I helped develop PGD so women could avoid genetic abortions. But it is now being used to avoid conditions that are consistent with good quality of life and even to select children of a specific gender or with other specific traits. PGD can even be used for cloning …

Dr. Staiman:

> Absolutely.

[refers to PowerPoint presentation]

> Look class how we divide this embryo into eight blastomeres that we can then be grown into eight identical embryos. This type of cloning is permitted in Canada, as long as we use the cloned embryos for stem cell research, rather than grow them into children —

Dr. Blume:

> I have another worry about PGD —

Dr. Staiman:

> I'm sure you do. But aren't you supposed to get into the fluff
> stuff this afternoon?

Dr. Blume:

> I worry that the money directed toward searching for genes
> for blonde hair, blue eyes, and other enhancements, is
> distracting scientists from research that could help, for
> example, children with muscular dystrophy walk again and
> live past their teens without having to be on ventilators for
> years and years. I'm sorry, Dr. Staiman, I know that you
> don't "worry" as much as I do.

Dr. Staiman:

> Actually, I don't "worry" at all. And as I've learned not
> to debate your misplaced passion, my friend, I will stick
> to the science where there can be no worries, because
> science is absolute.

Dr. Blume:

> Science is not absolute and a scientist's deadliest sin is
> certainty.

Dr. Staiman:

>Science is certain.

Dr. Blume:

>But its applications are not. Ask Einstein. It is arrogant for us to believe that in the future we will possess the silver sutures required to re-sew a society that we open to morally unexplored science today.

Dr. Staiman:

>Well, class, I wish we could continue this discussion, but as Dr. Blume and I have patients waiting, and you will soon have to get on to your next class, let's really stick to the science. It's all you need to know for your exams anyway.

[Dr. Blume exits.]

>All right. Here we see a —

[fade to women]

Scene 8

[Spot on Heather and Rose.]

Rose: Heather, I'm really sorry if I offended you.

Heather: You didn't offend me.

[tics]

Rose: But I can see that you're upset by what I said about Richard.

Heather:[*tics*]

It's not what you said about your brother.

Rose: Then what?

Heather: [*tics*]

It's just—

[gathers control]

it's just you can become pregnant at any time you want, and yet you choose to go through IVF

[tics]

with all the drugs, surgery, pain, money

[pauses]

to make sure your child won't be like

Rose: Richard?

[pauses]

But it's better than having a genetic abortion like in my

last pregnancy. The choice is that or PGD to prevent

having …

Heather: [*tics*]

A child like me?

[tics]

Rose: But I already told you I didn't know there was anything wrong

with you.

Heather: But now you know there is.

Rose: No I don't. I mean …

Heather: It's okay, Rose.

Rose: You're fine now.

Heather: And don't you think your child will be?

Rose: I can't forget how hard it was for Richard; how hard Richard

was for all of us.

[Music starts.]

Rose: I don't want that for Alan and me. Or for my child.

Song: I Just Want My Child to Be Normal

Rose:

Verse 1 I just want my child to be normal

It's my responsibility

I choose to use the key provided me

Verse 2 I just want my child to be normal

Why should it start with a disease?

When life's challenges, science can ease

Chorus If I don't do everything for my baby

If I don't remove the bad gene link

What will other people think of me

And my baby

I must do everything for my baby.

Verse 3: I just want my child to be normal

Why burden an innocent life

When science can prevent expected strife?

Verse 4: I just want my child to be normal

I see what lies in store

I've heard them laugh so loud through bolted doors

Bridge Life will always bring us challenges

To those even perfect at birth

So why add extra challenges

Why not benefit from all that science is worth

Removing bad genes is so easy now

They can do tests before you're pregnant now

They can make life so much easier now

We can all have all that we want.

Verse 5 I just want my child to be normal

I don't mean to offend

I know that that's the message that I send

I know that that's the message that I send

I just want my child to be normal

[Song ends.]

Rose: I'm sorry.

Heather: [*tics*]

It's okay. I suppose a lot of people share your point of view.

Rose: You know the difficulties that you've experienced and those around you have experienced. Why should anyone put a child through that, or go through that as a parent, when medical technology can prevent it? I mean for someone going through IVF like you, it's no extra medications or procedures—they just keep the embryos outside your body for two extra days and test them …

Heather: And put only the "normal" ones in my uterus.

Rose: Exactly.

[sees Heather's tics increase]

    Why does that bother you?

[Music starts. Heather struggles to gain control.]

Song: I Always Thought That I Was Normal

Heather: You see, Rose,

Verse 1   I always thought that I was normal

    Just burst out from time to time

    I always thought that I was normal

    My tics were just a problem of mine

Verse 2   I always thought that I was normal

    I have family, friends, and fun

    I always thought that I was normal

    Not a burden to anyone

Chorus: If 31 years ago they had PGD

    Would 31 years ago been kind to me

    Or would 31 years ago my mother have rejected me

    A lifetime of beauty I would not see

Verse 3 I always thought that I was normal

Though life had challenges for me

I could be anyone I wanted to be

A full member of society

Verse 4 I always thought that I was normal

That my life had love, had value

I always thought that I was normal

That I belong here as much as you

Chorus This lifetime of beauty never seen

[Rose and Heather sing the next two verses simultaneously.]

Rose: *[sings to the tune of I Just Want My Child to Be Normal]*

I just want my child to be normal

Why should it start with a disease?

When life's challenges, science can ease

Heather: *[sings simultaneously with Rose, to the tune of I Always Thought That I Was Normal]*

I always thought that I was normal

Just burst out from time to time

Life's challenges, I can handle with ease.

Heather: Think about your brother. Would you rather he had never

lived at all?

Rose: [*sings to the tune of I Just Want My Child to Be Normal*]

If I don't do everything for my baby

If I don't remove the bad gene link

What will people think of me and my baby

I must do everything for my baby

Heather: [*sings simultaneously with Rose, to the tune of I Always*

Thought That I Was Normal]

No one has the perfect baby

Don't remove the bad gene link

Who cares what people think of my baby

Everything for my baby

Scene 9

[Heather moves to a seat in the consultation room, stage left, where she is joined by Dr. Staiman. At stage right, the podium is replaced by two chairs to mirror the consultation room on stage left. Rose moves to a chair stage right, opposite Dr. Blume.]

Heather: [*hesitates*]

Dr. Staiman, your orchid pictures are beautiful.

Dr. Staiman:

[looks at Heather's chart]

I am really quite pleased with my flower family.

Heather: How do you make them so beautiful?

Dr. Staiman:

Genetic power creates perfect flowers.

Heather: [*masking manoeuvres*]

Genetic power?

Dr. Staiman:

I insert genes for brilliant colour and specially shaped petals.

Heather: [*masking manoeuvres*]

And the orchids with these genes, are they as healthy as natural orchids?

Dr. Staiman:

> There aren't many "natural" orchids anymore. And as
> genetically manipulated orchids all grow indoors, they can
> live a long time looking perfect, as long as their owners take
> good care of them.

[looks up]

> Your husband's not with you?

Heather: I'm sorry, he's working. We both can't afford to miss a day's
work while we're saving every cent for IVF.

Dr. Staiman:

> Yes. Canada's the only developed country that still doesn't
> cover IVF. The irony is that IVF would save the government
> money.

Heather: How?

Dr. Staiman:

> By avoiding high-order multiple pregnancies.

Heather: High order multiple …?

Dr. Staiman:

> You know, quadruplets, quintuplets. Taking fertility drugs
> without the protection of IVF has made Canada the world

leader in multiple pregnancies and in the resulting premature births that cause cognitive and physical damage to the children.

Heather: Oh.

Dr. Staiman:

Heather, I prefer to meet with couples together. It'll avoid interrogation when you go home, and help your husband be more supportive.

Heather: [*tics*]

Sean never interrogates me, and he's always supportive.

Dr. Staiman:

Okay, but there are issues that do involve your husband. You both have to sign the consent to freeze your extra embryos, and possibly donate some of them to stem cell research.

Heather: Freeze? Will my embryos be safe if you freeze them?

Dr. Staiman:

Absolutely. We've been freezing embryos for 20 years. To avoid multiple pregnancies, we only transfer a couple of embryos to your uterus during the treatment cycle. By freezing the rest of them, we give you a chance of becoming

347

pregnant because later we can transfer them to your uterus, one or two at a time, without you needing more fertility drugs and egg retrieval surgeries.

Heather: I see.

Dr. Staiman:

However, you may choose to donate a few of your extra embryos to stem cell research rather than freeze them.

Heather: Uh-huh.

Dr. Staiman:

And you and your husband will also have to decide on the disposition of your frozen embryos once you have as many children as you want.

Heather: Disposition?

Dr. Staiman:

Your options are stem cell research, donation to another infertile couple, or discard.

Heather: [*starts to speak but tics instead*]

Dr. Staiman, I guess you have the same passion to create perfect people as you do for creating perfect orchids.

Dr. Staiman:

> Perfect people?

Heather: You know, people without any flaws.

Dr. Staiman:

> I'm not looking to replicate my orchid research on people.

Heather: But you do test the genes of embryos before you put them in the woman's uterus?

Dr. Staiman:

> Preimplantation genetic diagnosis.

Heather: Yes.

Dr. Staiman:

> Aha, you've learned about PGD from that TV show on the little girl dying from Fanconi's anemia. Several patients have mentioned it.

Heather: What does testing embryos have to do with a girl dying?

Dr. Staiman:

> Testing embryos saved her life.

Heather: How?

Dr. Staiman:

> The girl's name was Molly. In order to save her, her mother underwent IVF and PGD to select an embryo that would become a baby who could be a stem cell donor for Molly. It only took three cycles to find the perfect embryo to be the donor and then have the embryo implant. But Molly's alive and well because of PGD. Incidentally, the press called her brother a "saviour sibling."

Heather: Oh. But that's not what I was asking about.

Dr. Staiman:

> Go ahead, then.

Heather: Do women with genetic conditions

[tics increase]

> need to have their genes tested before you perform IVF?

Scene 10

[Lights come up on Rose and Dr. Blume who mirror Heather and Dr. Staiman.]

Dr. Blume:

Your husband's not here today, Rose?

Rose: No, but he understood everything you explained in our last meeting, and he definitely wants to pursue PGD.

Dr. Blume:

And you, Rose? Are you really sure you want to undergo PGD?

Rose: Yes, I'm sure.

Dr. Blume:

Do you have any questions about the IVF medications or surgery?

Rose: No. I really do think you've explained both very well.

Dr. Blume:

You must have some questions…

Rose: Okay, besides Tourette's, how many genetic diseases can PGD diagnose?

Dr. Blume:

"Diseases."

[pauses]

I prefer "conditions."

Rose: Fine, "conditions."

Dr. Blume:

Well, as of today, there are approximately 350. Within the next few years, well it depends where the research funding is directed and how one defines "condition."

Rose: Fine.

Dr. Blume

Are you sure you don't have any questions regarding the risks of PGD?

Rose: You did say that you can take cells from my embryos without causing them any harm.

Dr. Blume:

Not exactly. Perhaps I said that PGD has only been used for a little more than 10 years, and so far the research suggests there is no increase in health problems in children who have undergone it as embryos, when compared to children of parents of similar age.

Rose: Then my child will be normal if you do PGD?

Dr. Blume:

I'm not sure what "normal" is, Rose. If you mean, will your child have Tourette Syndrome if we only implant embryos free of Tourette's gene markers,

[pauses]

likely not.

Rose: That's good.

Dr. Blume:

But even the embryos with markers for Tourette's may not exhibit any of the manifestations that you're worried about. And if your child has some challenges, you may be able to handle them very well.

Rose: You've told me this before.

Dr. Blume:

And remember, IVF has risks to your health. And discarding embryos with markers for Tourette's decreases your chance of IVF pregnancy by half. That makes it less than a 20%

chance each time you undergo the drugs and surgery. Rose, there is a significant chance that you may never become pregnant.

Rose: Look, you've already told me all this before, but you don't seem to understand that I'd rather have no child than a child like my brother. Alan and I could handle a childless marriage. We've got so many other things going in our lives.

[pauses]

So many things a child like Richard would disrupt.

[Lights fade.]

Scene 11

[Lights come up on Heather and Dr. Staiman.]

Dr. Staiman:

Heather, why are you so interested in genetic testing?

[reads chart]

You don't have any children yet, so I assume you're not going to request we use PGD for gender selection, which, incidentally, we won't do in this Clinic.

[Heather starts to speak but stops.]

Dr. Staiman:

But you know there's a finger-prick blood test you can buy to see if you're pregnant with a boy or a girl and you just mail it in to the states.

Heather: I don't care at all about the gender of my child.

Dr. Staiman:

Well you don't seem to be the enhancement type.

Heather: Enhancement?

[tics]

Dr. Staiman:

> Some of our patients purchase sperm from Nobel Laureate sperm banks, and some IVF clinics assist couples buying eggs from California models on Internet auctions. Are you okay, Heather?

Heather: Dr. Staiman, I don't want my child to have enhanced characteristics, but,

[pauses, tics increasing]

> there is something that runs in my family.

Dr. Staiman:

[looks at chart]

> There is.

Heather: I have Tourette Syndrome.

Dr. Staiman:

[looks puzzled at Heather, then again at her chart]

> But it doesn't say that in the questionnaire you filled in.

Heather: *[tics]*

> The questionnaire didn't ask about Tourette's.

Dr. Staiman:

[points to chart]

> It asked about medical problems.

Heather: [tics totally unmask]

> I never considered Tourette's

[tic]

> to be a medical problem.

Dr. Staiman:

> You don't?

Heather: [*tics*]

> No, I don't.

Dr. Staiman:

> Really.

[looks at chart]

> But you want to have PGD to avoid Tourette's?

Heather: No I don't.

Dr. Staiman:

> Then why are you so interested in PGD?

Heather: Because I was just talking to a woman in your waiting room, and now I'm worried that you won't let me have IVF if I didn't agree to PGD.

[tics are extreme]

Dr. Staiman:

We certainly do *not* insist that our IVF patients with genetic diseases have PGD.

[pauses]

Is there anything I can do to help you?

Heather: No. I just need a second to regain control.

[masking manoeuvres to fight tics]

Dr. Staiman:

I apologize for anything I may have said that is causing you to react this way. I—

Heather: It's not what you said.

Dr. Staiman:

What then?

Heather: You probably see me as an aberration that can be prevented by genetic technology.

Dr. Staiman:

> No. I—

Heather: A mutation that should not be passed on.

Dr. Staiman:

> Heather, I—

Heather: And that makes me feel guilty about not wanting to go through

> PGD for my child.

Dr. Staiman:

> I couldn't even tell that you have Tourette's.

Heather: It makes me feel like a bad mother,

[tics]

> before I'm even pregnant, because, actually I wouldn't mind

> if my child had Tourette's.

Dr. Staiman:

> I'm sure you will be a wonderful mother.

Heather: Don't patronize me.

Dr. Staiman:

> I… Let me assure you I will perform IVF on you without

> genetic testing.

Heather: [*pauses, then speaks slowly*]

> But you think I should go through PGD to avoid a child with Tourette's.

Dr. Staiman:

> It's up to you. You're right; discarding the Tourette's embryos would decrease your chance of pregnancy by half. And those embryos may not even exhibit the condition.

Heather: [*tics*]

> So then why would you help any woman have PGD for Tourette's?

[Dr. Staiman starts to speak but stops.]

> Please answer the question.

Dr. Staiman:

> I don't know. Because it's her choice. Perhaps she wants…

Heather: A perfect orchid?

Dr. Staiman:

> An orchid? I think my enthusiasm for orchids has confused your thinking.

Heather: My thinking?

Dr. Staiman:

>Let's talk about this again at your next visit. But I can tell you, it's completely your decision.

Heather: Thank you.

Dr. Staiman:

>Let's get your IVF blood work done now. We'll need that regardless of what you choose. The nurse will prepare all the requisition forms. I'm afraid it will take a while.

Heather: That's fine.

Dr. Staiman:

>Please take a seat in the waiting room.

Heather: Thank you.

Dr. Staiman:

>Do you remember the way back? The corridors are confusing here.

Heather: It's not the corridors that are confusing here.

[Heather exits. Dr. Staiman looks puzzled and remains stationary on stage during next scene. Lights fade.]

Scene 12

[Lights come up on Rose and Dr. Blume.]

Dr. Blume:

> I appreciate that, Rose, but are you sure that you want to
> go through all the medications and surgery?

Rose: Why do you keep asking me that? I've already told you:

> absolutely, yes!

Dr. Blume:

> Is something troubling you Rose?

Rose: You seem to think I'm over-reacting by going through with this.

Dr. Blume:

> I can't put myself in your position.

Rose: You're being evasive. Let me ask you directly. Would you

> want your wife to have PGD to avoid a child with
>
> Tourette Syndrome?

Dr. Blume:

> It's not appropriate for doctors to answer questions like
>
> that. As your doctor I'm only here to help you do what
>
> you want to do.

Rose: Then support me in my decision!

Dr. Blume:

> I'm sorry if it appears that I'm not supporting you, but
> it's my obligation as your physician to caution you
> regarding the risks of PGD.

Rose: Risks to me? Risks to my child? Risks to whom?

Dr. Blume:

> Well —

[starts to speak and stops]

Rose: Just help me have PGD and stop making me feel guilty about
          being here.

Dr. Blume:

> I … That's the last thing a physician —

Rose: Perhaps Dr. Staiman would be more supportive. Can I see him?

Dr. Blume:

> I will certainly refer you to Dr. Staiman if you wish. But
> I —

Rose: I must have PGD for both Alan and my child. And if *I* have
          PGD, my children won't have to, and their children
          won't have Tourette's.

Dr. Blume:

[pauses]

> I really want to discuss this further, but I have 150 students
> waiting for me. I can be back here in an hour. Please, Rose,
> if it's not too inconvenient, will you allow me the
> opportunity to speak with you? Please go down to the lab for
> the PGD blood work, and come back afterwards. Please.

Rose: Okay, I'll come back. I *am* a bit confused. And I wasn't when
   I came here this morning.

Dr. Blume:

[Dr. Blume's eyes follow Rose as she exits.]

> I'm confused too, Rose.

Song: Guilty

*[During the song, Dr. Blume "travels" from his office to the lecture
hall.]*

Dr. Blume:

Verse 1 Why can't I be what you have a right to expect?

   Why can't I give your decision that respect?

   Why can't I provide support and competence?

   Why do I steal your dignity and your confidence?

Verse 2 Instead of helping you pursue what you choose

I worry about what others, and what they could lose

Why do I stand in the way of your choice?

Where's my compassion, I'm not hearing your voice?

Chorus I'm guilty for my role in this technology

Without concern for where it may lead

And now I've made her feel guilty

Please forgive me.

Verse 3 For years I've taught what a good doctor should be

But I don't apply what I teach to me I tell you to be there for

each patient you serve Yet I deny her the care that all patients

deserve

Chorus I'm guilty for my role in this technology

Without concern for where it may lead

And now I've made her feel guilty

Please forgive me.

Verse 4 Caring for my patients, it's at the heart of me

How can I give up the biggest part of me?

How can I stay, how can I go?

If I can't give good care, how can I keep up this show?

[Dr. Blume stops singing, walks to lectern and speaks to class.]

Dr Blume:

> A good doctor must always help each patient pursue the treatment options available to her, cautioning her regarding the risks of medications and surgery, but ultimately supporting her in her decision. A good doctor must never allow personal concern, or even concern for others, to cloud the obligation to assist the patient in her choice. Okay class, back to the ethics of PGD.

[Lights up on Dr. Staiman. Dr. Staiman turns and looks at Dr. Blume.]

> Genetic technologies may lead to diversity's demise, may open the door to elitism and close the door on compassion. Are we creating a society that affords the rich the design of their child while we create a world that denies disabled persons dignity because they're different? Will educational and social support be excluded for children whose mothers choose not to access genetic testing? How will disabled people see themselves in genetic technology's magic mirror? We need to explore where science is leading us before we sentence our children to a world we won't know.

[Dr. Staiman walks over to Dr. Blume.]

366

In closing, let's look to the arts to illustrate our humanity. Walt Whitman praised the human body when he wrote "I sing the body *electric*." We should also sing the body *eclectic*, and praise the many variations of our humanness. Consider the magnificent canvasses by the French painter Seurat. His millions of tiny dots of paint, that vary in colour and size, and number per centimetre, create pictures of such splendour. Well, I see humanity as a magnificent canvas with each of us a very important dot, diverse in so many ways.

Dr. Staiman:

Dr. Blume ... if I might be allowed to add something.

Dr. Blume:

Well, I —

Dr. Staiman:

A good doctor must continue to learn from his patients and his colleagues. In support of Dr. Blume's thinking, let me share my experience with orchids. The most powerful moment at an orchid show is the first image you see when you walk into the exhibit hall: that all-encompassing picture of diverse colour and configuration. Each orchid is but a tiny dot in the room. Each perfection of petal and colour is truly inconsequential, it's all beautiful.

Scene 13

[Heather and Rose enter the waiting room from opposite sides. They face each other with the four chairs between them, their eyes diverted from each other until Rose speaks.]

Rose: Heather ... I really am sorry if I offended you.

Heather: *[tics]*

        You didn't offend me.

Rose: I really am sorry.

[uncomfortable silence]

        What's Dr. Staiman like?

[another uncomfortable silence]

        Was he supportive?

Heather: Did you ...

[tics]

        did you discuss PGD with Dr. Blume?

Rose: Yes.

Heather: *[pauses]*

        Are you going to have it?

Rose: Yes, Heather.

Heather: I see.

Rose: Are you considering having it too?

Heather: [*tics*]

Now you're offending me

[tics]

and my parents.

Rose: Your parents?

Heather: No matter how many times my parents were asked to take me out of a restaurant because of my unusual behaviour, they were never upset with me. Just the opposite. They would encourage me with "Let's try another restaurant in a few weeks."

Rose: That's your experience.

Heather: Yes it is. My parents loved me. And their love taught me to love. And I will love my child no matter what.

Rose: It's not that simple.

Heather: I think it is.

Rose: I told Alan before we married about the gene that runs in my family and he said it wasn't a problem. But I know he doesn't want it to run in *his* family. My brother's doing just fine now. He's an auto mechanic. I can't do Richard to Alan.

[pauses]

369

Alan needs normal. He's never gone through adversity, does not understand adversity, need not understand adversity.

Heather: Adversity? Yes, I had challenges when I was a kid. And, as you can see, I still do. But we all have challenges, or will. You said that yourself.

Rose: Heather, not everyone has your strength.

Heather: Maybe you do.

Rose: I know I don't.

[pauses]

I'm not you, Heather. I wish I were more like you.

Heather: No you don't.

Rose: I do.

Heather: Then why are you having PGD to prevent someone like me from being born?

Rose: That's not it.

[pauses]

Anyway, why are you so upset with me when we're both choosing what we want?

Heather: Because your choice steals something from me.

Rose: Steals what?

370

Heather: I don't know exactly. Maybe my right to exist? Maybe my

right to have a child without guaranteeing …

[works hard to control tics]

Maybe —

Rose: But, I don't want to have another genetic abortion —

Heather: *[tics]*

Or a child like me.

Rose: Can't you see I would be less of a mother if my child's life

was less than it could be. Less of a wife if my husband's

life was less than it could be.

Heather: Less? Are you saying I'm less of a person than you? Are you

saying that I'm not as responsible as you?

Rose: Heather, if an inherited disease can*not* be prevented, that's one

thing. But when it can… Can't you see that when genetic

science offers me a solution I have no choice but to choose

it. Can't you see that Heather?

Heather: *[tics]*

No. I can't allow myself to go there.

[Blackout.]

Scene 14

[Lights go up on the long laboratory bench and the semi-robotic motion of the lab techs.]

Song: Embryo Engineers refrain

Verse 1: We are good lifeguards

      Care for our kids

      Help them swim

      Lives begin

      Beneath glass lids

Verse 2: Trained to be cogs

      In this machine

      Holding hopes

      In microscopes

      Fulfilling dreams

Chorus: Science blessed

      Happiness

      Proud to be

      Embryo engineers

      Science blessed

      Happiness

      Proud to be

Embryo engineers

Embryo engineers

[Blackout.]

FINIS

Acknowledgements

I would like to thank Liza Balkan and Rebecca Cann for their dramaturgy of the 2005-2006 remounting of *Orchids,* and Robert Richardson, Marquis Entertainment Inc., Toronto for producing the national tour. Canadian Institutes of Health Research and Health Canada contributed significant funding to this tour. I would like to thank Professor Susan Cox, University of British Columbia, for helping me achieve this funding and the analysis of *Orchids* and audience member comments as Canada's first citizen deliberation using theatre for health policy development. I would also like to thank Louise Fagan for her contributions to the original production

Portions of *Orchids* were published in *Mappa Mundi: Mapping Culture/Mapping the World* University of Windsor Press J. Murray (Ed).[46]

Score by Allyson Koffman, Steve Hardy, and Michael Barber, available from jeff.nisker@lhsc.on.ca.

---

[46] J.A. Nisker, Orchids: Not Necessarily A Gospel, In: Murray J, editors. Mappa Mundi: Mapping Culture/Mapping the World, University of Windsor Press, 2001, pp. 61-110.

Iguana Books

iguanabooks.com

If you enjoyed *From Calcedonies to Orchids: Plays Promoting Humanity in Health Policy* ...

Look for other books coming soon from Iguana Books! Subscribe to our blog for updates as they happen.

iguanabooks.com/blog/

You can also learn more about Jeff Nisker and his upcoming work on his blog.

jeffnisker.iguanabooks.com

If you're a writer ...

Iguana Books is always looking for great new writers, in every genre. We produce primarily ebooks but, as you can see, we do the occasional print book as well. Visit us at iguanabooks.com to see what Iguana Books has to offer both emerging and established authors.

iguanabooks.com/publishing-with-iguana/

If you're looking for another good book ...

All Iguana Books books are available on our website. We pride ourselves on making sure that every Iguana book is a great read.

iguanabooks.com/bookstore/

Visit our bookstore today and support your favourite author.

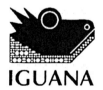

IGUANA

CPSIA information can be obtained at www.ICGtesting.com
Printed in the USA
LVOW07s0558011013

354780LV00008B/34/P